Myopericardial Diseases

Myocardial Diseases

Massimo Imazio

Myopericardial Diseases

Diagnosis and Management

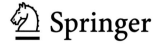 Springer

Massimo Imazio
Cardiology Department
Maria Vittoria Hospital
and Department of Public Health and Pediatrics
University of Torino
Torino
Italy

ISBN 978-3-319-27154-5   ISBN 978-3-319-27156-9   (eBook)
DOI 10.1007/978-3-319-27156-9

Library of Congress Control Number: 2015960845

Springer Cham Heidelberg New York Dordrecht London

Printed on acid-free paper

Springer International Publishing AG Switzerland is part of Springer Science+Business Media
(www.springer.com)

Preface

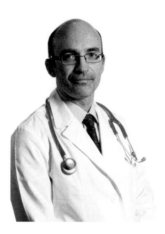

Pericardial diseases have been the "Cinderella" of heart diseases for decades. They have been poorly understood and studied even in medical schools, but they are not so uncommon in clinical practice, usually affecting young patients and having potential deep impact in their lives.

Unfortunately, there is limited knowledge on the pathogenesis of these diseases, and management has been mainly empirical before the first clinical trials and large prospective studies in the last 5–10 years. These diseases are often the manifestation of a systemic disease or a primary disease with pericardial or myopericardial involvement, and different medical specialties may be involved (e.g. cardiology, cardiac surgery, internal medicine, nephrology, rheumatology, clinical immunology, oncology), thus further complicating the diagnostic evaluation and subsequent management.

Moreover, the diagnosis of pericardial diseases is often challenging because symptoms and signs may be vague, insidious and non-specific, as well as findings from traditional diagnostic methods, such as ECG and chest x-ray.

It is so not surprising that the coping with these diseases may be especially difficult for practitioners and physicians.

On this basis, the aim of the present book is to provide a concise, updated, comprehensive review on the available data on the aetiology, diagnosis, therapy and prognosis of pericardial and myopericardial diseases with a special emphasis on practical management issues for clinical practice.

The format of each chapter is especially thought to be helpful in clinical practice, providing simple and straightforward indications and management issues that are based on updated research data and consistent and reviewed according to the most recent guidelines.

The reference section is structured especially to provide suggested readings for those interested to have in-depth views on a specific topic, including essentially only more recent publications limited to the last 5–10 years.

Last but not least, I would like to thank my mentors in Pericardiology, Professors Ralph Shabetai and David Spodick, Professor Lucia Mangiardi and my past Director Rita Trinchero, who gave me the task to develop and improve the management of pericardial diseases in my institution and supported me in my clinical and research activities. I am also thankful for their support to Dr Riccardo Belli and all the staff of the Cardiology Department of the Maria Vittoria Hospital who helped me in my research and clinical activities and especially Mrs Mara Carraro who assisted me in the ambulatory and day hospital activities dedicated to patients with myopericardial diseases.

I would like also to thank the editor for the support and give special thanks to my wife Silvia and children Marco, Luisa and Andrea who have always tolerated my hectic dedication to the study of myopericardial diseases and who know that I will always be there for them, although with pen in hand.

Torino, Italy   Massimo Imazio

Contents

Part III Specific Populations, Guidelines, Conclusions and Perspectives

Part I

General Evaluation of Myopericardial Diseases

Essential Anatomy and Physiology of the Pericardium for Clinical Practice

1

1.1 Anatomy of the Pericardium

The *pericardium* (from the Greek περί, "around", and κάρδιον, "heart") is a double-walled sac containing the heart and the roots of the great vessels. The pericardium is the external layer of the heart providing protection and support to inner structures. It is composed by and external fibroserosal part (parietal pericardium) and an internal serosal part (visceral pericardium) (Fig. 1.1). The internal serosal is also named epicardium, which has direct connection with the myocardium. The parietal pericardium has an inner serosal part that is in continuity with the epicardium and an external fibrous part (Fig. 1.2).

Between the visceral and parietal pericardial layers, a virtual pericardial cavity is filled by 20–30 ml of plasma ultrafiltrate (pericardial fluid) that acts as a lubricant allowing myocardial contraction without attrition with the surrounding anatomical structures [1, 2]. The pericardial fluid is produced by the serosal part of the pericardium which is provided by mesothelial cells with microvilla and cilia that further expand the available pericardial surface. The reflection of the visceral pericardium into the parietal pericardium over the great vessels is responsible for the creation of spaces, where pericardial fluid can accumulate and they can be seen on imaging. Greater spaces are called *sinuses*, while smaller spaces between adjacent anatomic structures are called *recesses*. The main sinuses include the *transverse sinus* located between the aorta and pulmonary trunk anteriorly and the atria and veins posteriorly and the *oblique sinus* located behind the left atrium and between the pulmonary veins and the inferior vena cava (Fig. 1.3) [3, 4].

Both sinuses may be accessed for electrophysiology purposes for ablation of cardiac arrhythmias. Fat is present under the epicardium (epicardial fat) and in connection with the parietal pericardium. Fat tissue provides mechanical, immunological protection of the heart, as well as a source of fatty acids and thus energy and may also have endocrine functions by cytokines that act through paracrine mechanisms on myocardial and endocardial cells [5].

© Springer International Publishing Switzerland 2016

M. Imazio, *Myopericardial Diseases: Diagnosis and Management*,

DOI 10.1007/978-3-319-27156-9_1

Fig. 1.1 The pericardium and the external envelope of the heart (see text for explanation) (Reproduced from Blausen.com staff, "Blausen gallery 2014", *Wikiversity Journal of Medicine* (licensed under CC BY 3.0))

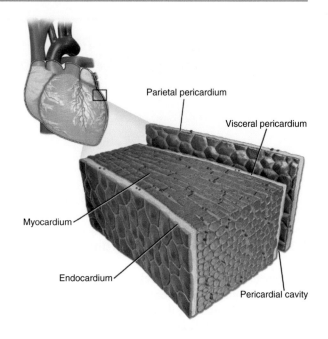

Fig. 1.2 Pericardial layers and cavity (Reproduced from *Anatomy & Physiology*, Connexions Web site. http://cnx.org/content/col11496/1.6/, 19 June 2013 (licensed under CC BY 3.0))

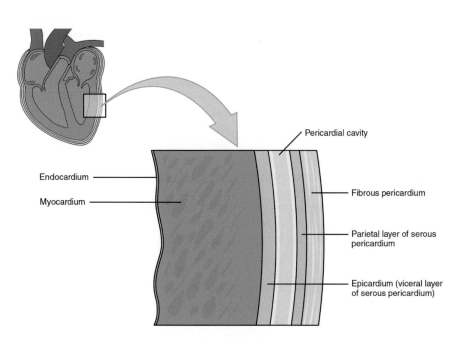

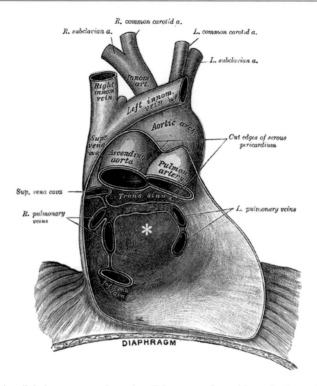

Fig. 1.3 Pericardial sinuses are main pericardial recesses formed by reflections of the pericardium over vascular and cardiac structures. The *transverse sinus* is between the aorta, pulmonary trunk and the atria and pulmonary veins. The oblique sinus (*) is posterior to the left atrium and between the inferior vena cava and pulmonary veins (From Henry Gray (1918) *Anatomy of the human body* (Bartleby.com: Gray's Anatomy, Plate 489), drawing in the public domain)

The pericardium is fixed to the surrounding anatomical structures by ligaments: anteriorly to sternum by the sternopericardial ligaments, posteriorly to the vertebral column and inferiorly to the diaphragm.

The normal thickness of the pericardium is less than 3 mm in imaging studies from clinical practice. In imaging the measure is overestimated and autoptic and surgical studies provide an anatomical size of less than 1–2 mm [4, 6].

The pericardium has an extensive network of lymphatics that drain substances from pericardial space and allow the spread of pathological process from and to the pericardium in case of mediastinal and pulmonary pathology. The anterior part of the pericardium is drained either upwards to anterior mediastinal lymph nodes or downwards to the diaphragm, the posterior part drains into paraesophageal and tracheobronchial lymph nodes and the inferior part into prepericardial, lateropericardial, paraesophageal and tracheobronchial lymph nodes, while the lateral parts drain into mediastinal, tracheobronchial, lateropericardial, prepericardial and paraesophageal lymph nodes (Fig. 1.4).

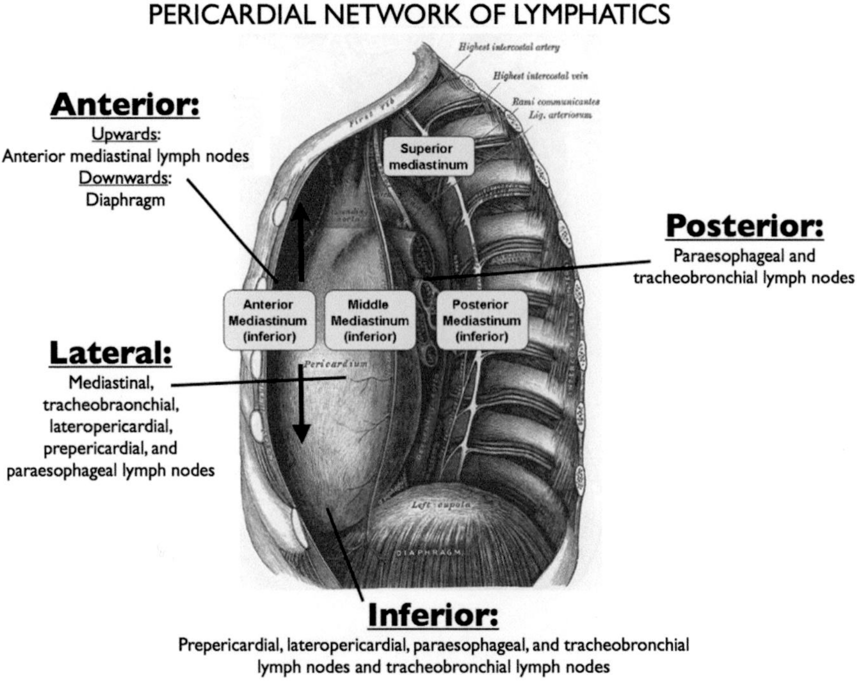

PERICARDIAL NETWORK OF LYMPHATICS

Anterior:
Upwards:
Anterior mediastinal lymph nodes
Downwards:
Diaphragm

Posterior:
Paraesophageal and
tracheobronchial lymph nodes

Lateral:
Mediastinal,
tracheobraonchial,
lateropericardial,
prepericardial, and
paraesophageal lymph nodes

Inferior:
Prepericardial, lateropericardial, paraesophageal, and tracheobronchial
lymph nodes and tracheobronchial lymph nodes

Fig. 1.4 The pericardial network of lymphatics. There are four main regions: anterior, posterior, inferior and lateral parts (Modified from Henry Gray (1918) *Anatomy of the human body*, drawing in the public domain)

The arterial blood supply of the pericardium is provided by the descending aorta, branches of the mammary arteries and musculophrenic arteries.

The pericardium has both a sympathetic (first dorsal ganglion, stellate ganglion, aortic and cardiac plexuses) and parasympathetic innervation (vagus, left recurrent laryngeal nerve, oesophageal plexus) [4].

1.2   Physiology of the Pericardium

The pericardium acts as a relatively inelastic sac, because of its high content of collagen fibres, enveloping the heart and providing mechanical protection to the heart allowing movement of cardiac chambers without attrition and also limiting their distension. This effect is especially evident on the right cardiac chambers.

This effect explains the exaggerated interventricular interdependence that can be observed in pathological conditions (e.g. cardiac tamponade and constrictive pericarditis), as well as how rapidly accumulating pericardial fluid may be responsible of cardiac tamponade with limited amount of fluid, such as 200–300 mL in

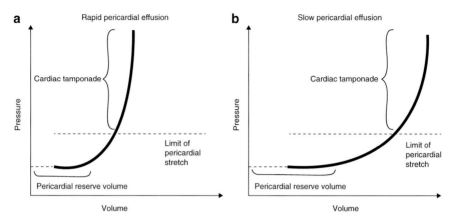

Fig. 1.5 Pressure/volume curve of the pericardium. The pericardium acts as a rather inelastic sac due to its high content of collagen fibres. On this basis, rapid changes of the volume of the pericardial space will reach soon the limit of pericardial stretch with a sudden rise of intrapericardial pressure (this explains the quick development of cardiac tamponade in these settings: e.g. aortic dissection with haemopericardium). On the contrary, slowly accumulating pericardial fluid can reach high volumes as high as 1–2 L without the development of cardiac tamponade (e.g. idiopathic chronic pericardial effusions) (Reproduced with permission from [6])

Table 1.1 Physiologic functions of the pericardium
Mechanical functions
Reduction of the attrition between the myocardium and surrounding structures
Limitation of the distension of cardiac chambers
Limitation of the regurgitation of cardiac valves
Barrier to mechanical and infections noxa
Immunological and additional functions
Protection from infectious agents
Production of factors that modulate sympathetic tone
Endocrine and metabolic functions of the epicardial fat
Fibrinolytic activity of pericardial mesothelial cells
Lymphatic drainage of the heart

haemopericardium. On the contrary, slowly accumulating pericardial fluid can allow the generation of large pericardial effusions as 1–2 L without the development of cardiac tamponade (e.g. large chronic pericardial effusions). This is well explained by the pressure-volume curve of the pericardium (Fig. 1.5) [6].

The pericardium is not simply a mechanical barrier but has also an active immunological role that is very relevant in inflammatory conditions, such as pericarditis and myocarditis.

Although the pericardium has several important functions (Table 1.1), its absence (total agenesis) or surgical removal (e.g. pericardiectomy) has limited consequences for life, and it is absolutely compatible with a normal life [1, 4].

Key Points
- The pericardium is composed by an outer parietal fibroserosal layer (*parietal pericardium*) and an inner serosal visceral layer (*visceral pericardium or epicardium*).
- A pericardial space is contained within the two layers and filled by 20–30 mL of plasma ultrafiltrate (*pericardial fluid*).
- The pericardium acts as a rather inelastic sac surrounding and protecting the heart allowing myocardial contraction without attrition and regulating the expansion of cardiac chamber.
- The pericardium is rather stiff: this means that is not able to fit rapid changes of volume without a sudden increase of intrapericardial pressure: this leads to cardiac tamponade for small quickly increasing pericardial effusions but also allow the formation of a large slowly accumulating pericardial effusion, such as a chronic idiopathic pericardial effusion.
- Additional functions include immune, metabolic and endocrine functions that are emerging properties of the pericardium.

References

1. Little WC, Freeman GL. Pericardial diseases. Circulation. 2006;113:1622–32.
2. LeWinter MM. Clinical practice. Acute pericarditis. N Engl J Med. 2014;371:2410–6.
3. Lachman N, Syed FF, Habib A, Kapa S, Bisco SE, Venkatachalam KL, Asirvatham SJ. Correlative anatomy for the electrophysiologist, part I: the pericardial space, oblique sinus, transverse sinus. J Cardiovasc Electrophysiol. 2010;21:1421–6.
4. Peebles CR, Shambrook JS, Harden SP. Pericardial disease – anatomy and function. Br J Radiol. 2011;84 Spec No 3:S324–37.
5. Bertaso AG, Bertol D, Duncan BB, Foppa M. Epicardial fat: definition, measurements and systematic review of main outcomes. Arq Bras Cardiol. 2013;101:e18–28.
6. Imazio M, Adler Y. Management of pericardial effusion. Eur Heart J. 2013;34:1186–97.

Aetiology and Classification of Pericardial Diseases

2

2.1   Overview and Epidemiology

The pericardium may be affected by all kinds of aetiological agents, although specific aetiologies are much more common in clinical practice and may have specific regional changes according to the prevalence of infectious diseases, especially tuberculosis (Table 2.1) [1–9].

The pericardial may be affected alone or be involved in a systemic disease or a localization of another pathological process affecting primarily another organ or tissue.

Tuberculosis is the major cause of pericardial diseases all over the world being the most common aetiology in countries with a high prevalence of tuberculosis, such as developing countries (Fig. 2.1) [2, 3, 6, 8].

A high prevalence (>60 % of cases) has been reported in sub-Saharan Africa, and tuberculous pericarditis is especially associated with HIV infection in these settings [6]. On the contrary, tuberculous aetiology accounts for less than 5 % of cases in developed countries, such as Western Europe and North America, where there is a low prevalence of tuberculosis [2–4, 7]. In these countries, most cases are labelled to be "idiopathic" and are presumed to be viral in most cases (>85 %). The epidemiological background is essential to develop a rational, cost-effective, diagnostic evaluation since the aetiology search should be especially focused to exclude major aetiologies in order to avoid many diagnostic tests with a very limited diagnostic yield [2–5, 9]. Immigration may change the current aetiological spectrum in the next few years, and thus a careful consideration of these aspects as well as ethnic issues is warranted.

A simple and commonly used classification divides pericardial aetiologies into infectious and non-infectious (Table 2.2).

There are limited epidemiological data on pericardial and myopericardial diseases. The incidence of acute pericarditis has been reported as 27.7 cases per 100.000 population/year in an Italian urban area (North Italy) with concomitant myocarditis in about 15 % of these cases [10].

© Springer International Publishing Switzerland 2016   9
M. Imazio, *Myopericardial Diseases: Diagnosis and Management*,
DOI 10.1007/978-3-319-27156-9_2

Table 2.1 Aetiology of pericarditis in major reported published series

Aetiology	Reported frequency (%)
Idiopathic	15 % (Africa) to 80–90 % (Europe)
Infectious pericarditis	
Viral (e.g. *Coxsackie*, EBV, CMV, HIV, *Parvovirus* B 19)	Largely unknown (30–50 % in Marburg experience, Germany)
Bacterial:	
Tuberculosis	1–4 % (Italy, Spain, France), up to 70 % (Africa)
Purulent	<1 % (Europe) to 2–3 % (Africa)
Other infectious causes	Rare (largely unknown)
Non-infectious pericarditis	
Neoplastic aetiology	5–9–35 % (in tertiary European referral centres)
Autoimmune*	2–24 %
Other infectious causes	Rare (largely unknown)

* including systemic inflammatory diseases and post-cardiac injury syndromes

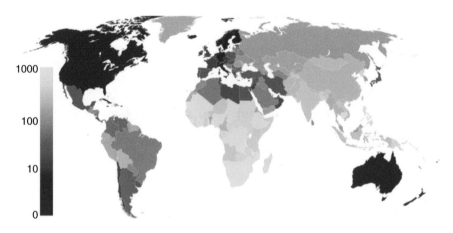

Fig. 2.1 Prevalence of tuberculosis per 100,000 people is highest in sub-Saharan Africa, and it is also relatively high in Asia. From Wikipedia, with data from the World Health Organization (2009) Global tuberculosis control: epidemiology, strategy, financing (image in the public domain)

Pericarditis is responsible of 0.1 % of all hospital admissions and 5 % of emergency room admissions for chest pain [2, 3]. Data collected from a Finnish national registry (2000–2009) showed a standardized incidence rate of hospitalizations for acute pericarditis of 3.32 per 100.000 person-years. Men aged 16–65 were at higher risk for pericarditis (relative risk 2.02) with the highest-risk difference among young adults compared to the overall population. Acute pericarditis caused 0.20 % of all cardiovascular admissions. The proportion of caused admissions declined in younger patients. In-hospital mortality rate for acute pericarditis was 1.1 % and was increased with age and severe co-infections (pneumonia or septicaemia) [11]. Recurrences of pericarditis are common and may affect about one third of cases

Table 2.2 Main aetiologies of pericardial diseases. A simple classification is to divide into infectious and non-infectious causes

Infectious causes
Viral (common): enteroviruses (coxsackie viruses, echoviruses), herpesviruses (EBV, CMV, HHV-6), adenoviruses, parvovirus B19 (possible overlap with aetiologic viral agents of myocarditis)
Bacterial: *Mycobacterium tuberculosis* (common, other bacterial rare), *Coxiella burnetii*, Borrelia burgdorferi, rarely – *Pneumococcus* spp., *Meningococcus* spp., *Gonococcus* spp., *Streptococcus* spp., *Staphylococcus* spp., *Haemophilus* spp., *Chlamydia* spp., *Mycoplasma* spp., *Legionella* spp., *Leptospira* spp., *Listeria* spp., *Providencia stuartii*
Fungal (very rare): *Histoplasma* spp. (more likely in immunocompetent patients), *Aspergillus* spp., *Blastomyces* spp., *Candida* spp. (more likely in immunocompromised host)
Parasitic (very rare): *Echinococcus* spp., *Toxoplasma* spp.
Non-infectious causes
Autoimmune (common):
Systemic autoimmune and auto-inflammatory diseases (systemic lupus erythematosus, Sjögren syndrome, rheumatoid arthritis, scleroderma), systemic vasculitides (i.e.: eosinophilic granulomatosis with polyangiitis or allergic granulomatosis, previously named Churg-Strauss syndrome, Horton disease, Takayasu disease, Behçet syndrome), sarcoidosis, familial Mediterranean fever, inflammatory bowel diseases, Still disease
Neoplastic:
Primary tumours (rare, above all pericardial mesothelioma)
Secondary metastatic tumours (common, above all lung and breast cancer, lymphoma)
Metabolic:
Uremia, myxedema, anorexia nervosa, other rare
Traumatic and Iatrogenic:
Early onset (rare):
Direct injury (penetrating thoracic injury, oesophageal perforation)
Indirect injury (non-penetrating thoracic injury, radiation injury)
Delayed onset:
Pericardial injury syndromes (common) postmyocardial infarction syndrome, postpericardiotomy syndrome, post-traumatic, including forms after iatrogenic trauma (e.g. coronary percutaneous intervention, pacemaker lead insertion and radiofrequency ablation)
Drug-related (rare):
Lupus-like syndrome (procainamide, hydralazine, methyldopa, isoniazid, phenytoin);
Antineoplastic drugs (often associated with a cardiomyopathy, may cause a pericardiopathy): doxorubicin and daunorubicin, cytosine arabinoside, 5-fluorouracil, cyclophosphamide
Hypersensitivity pericarditis with eosinophilia: penicillins, amiodarone, methysergide, mesalazine, clozapine, minoxidil, dantrolene, practolol, phenylbutazone, thiazides, streptomycin, thiouracils, streptokinase, p-aminosalicylic acid, sulfa drugs, cyclosporine, bromocriptine, several vaccines, GM-CSF, anti-TNF agents
Other (common): amyloidosis, aortic dissection, pulmonary arterial hypertension and chronic heart failure

Modified from [1, 2, 9]
spp. species

after a first episode of acute pericarditis not treated with colchicine and even up to 50 % of cases after a first recurrence [12–15].

2.2 Infectious Aetiologies

In developed countries with a low prevalence of tuberculosis, viral infections are presumed to be the most common causes of pericardial diseases [1–4, 9]. Pericarditis with or without pericardial effusion is the most common form of pericardial disease. Often preceded by a flu-like syndromes or gastroenteritis, pericarditis follows after few weeks the initial viral illness. A definite diagnosis would require the detection of viral genome in pericardial fluid or tissue, but this is generally not sough and even necessary in clinical practice due to the usual benign and self-limiting course of the disease. Viral serology and culture from swabs do not provide reliable results and only suggest the presence of a recent viral infection without demonstrating a pericardial localization. In any case, it should be remarked that even when identified, a viral aetiology does not change the management, since there are no proven treatments to offer to immunocompetent patients [9, 16].

Other bacterial causes beyond tuberculosis are rare. Purulent pericarditis is quite rare in the antibiotic era as well as in immunocompetent patients [3, 9].

2.3 Non-infectious Aetiologies

The most common non-infectious aetiologies include systemic inflammatory diseases and post-cardiac injury syndromes (overall about 5–24 % of all cases in developed countries) and metastatic involvement of the pericardium, especially in lung cancer, breast cancer and lymphomas and leukaemias (overall another 5–10 % of all cases) [16–20]. Other causes are not common and should be suspected according to specific histories and clinical presentations that will be detailed and reviewed in the following chapters.

2.4 Pericardial Syndromes

Pericardial syndromes include different clinical presentations of pericardial diseases with a more or less specific signs and symptoms (Fig. 2.2).

The main pericardial syndromes include:

1. Pericarditis with or without pericardial effusion (very common)
2. Pericarditis with myocarditis (myopericarditis and perimyocarditis)
3. Pericardial effusion (common)
4. Cardiac tamponade (often)
5. Constrictive pericarditis (rare)
6. Pericardial masses and cysts (relatively rare)

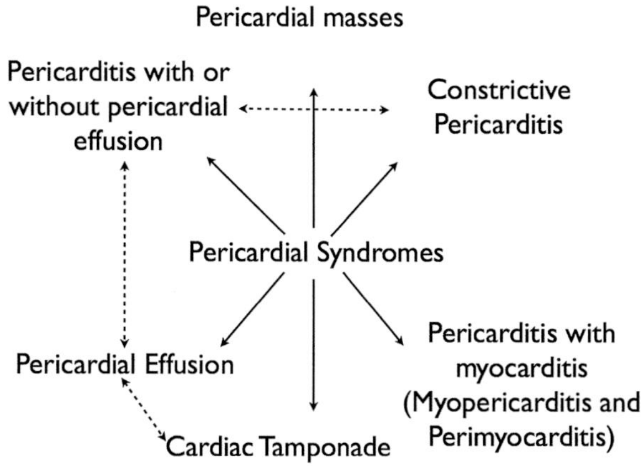

Pericardial masses

Pericarditis with or without pericardial effusion

Constrictive Pericarditis

Pericardial Syndromes

Pericardial Effusion

Pericarditis with myocarditis (Myopericarditis and Perimyocarditis)

Cardiac Tamponade

Fig. 2.2 The main pericardial syndromes include pericarditis, pericardial effusion, cardiac tamponade, constrictive pericarditis and pericardial masses. Some of them may evolve into another (e.g. pericardial effusion and cardiac tamponade, pericarditis and constrictive pericarditis)

A detailed description of each syndrome will be provided in the following chapters with a focus on diagnosis, clinical management, therapy and prognosis for clinical practice.

Key Points
- The pericardium may be affected as an isolated process or as part of a systemic disease or as a consequence of a pericardial localization of a disease of another organ/tissue (e.g. lung cancer).
- There are several potential possible aetiologies, usually divided into infectious and non-infectious.
- Overall, the main cause of pericardial diseases is tuberculosis considering developing countries with a high prevalence of tuberculosis.
- In developed countries (with a low prevalence of tuberculosis), the most common aetiologies are presumed to be viral, immune-mediated forms (systemic inflammatory diseases, post-cardiac injury syndromes) and cancer.
- In clinical practice, there are few usual presentations with distinctive signs and symptoms that are usually named pericardial syndromes: pericarditis with or without pericardial effusion (very common), pericarditis with myocarditis (common), isolated pericardial effusion (common), cardiac tamponade (often), constrictive pericarditis (rare), pericardial masses and cysts.

References

1. Imazio M. Contemporary management of pericardial diseases. Curr Opin Cardiol. 2012;27:308–17.
2. Imazio M, Gaita F. Diagnosis and treatment of pericarditis. Heart. 2015;101:1159–68.
3. Imazio M, Gaita F, LeWinter M. Evaluation and treatment of pericarditis: a systematic review. JAMA. 2015;314:1498–506.
4. Imazio M, Spodick DH, Brucato A, Trinchero R, Adler Y. Controversial issues in the management of pericardial diseases. Circulation. 2010;121:916–28.
5. Permanyer-Miralda G. Acute pericardial disease: approach to the aetiologic diagnosis. Heart. 2004;90:252–4.
6. Mayosi BM. Contemporary trends in the epidemiology and management of cardiomyopathy and pericarditis in sub-Saharan Africa. Heart. 2007;93:1176–83.
7. Gouriet F, Levy PY, Casalta JP, Zandotti C, Collart F, Lepidi H, Cautela J, Bonnet JL, Thuny F, Habib G, Raoult D. Etiology of pericarditis in a prospective cohort of 1162 cases. Am J Med. 2015;128:784.e1–8.
8. Sliwa K, Mocumbi AO. Forgotten cardiovascular diseases in Africa. Clin Res Cardiol. 2010;99:65–74.
9. Adler Y, Charron P, Imazio M, Badano L, Barón-Esquivias G, Bogaert J, Brucato A, Gueret P, Klingel K, Lionis C, Maisch B, Mayosi B, Pavie A, Ristić AD, Sabaté Tenas M, Seferovic P, Swedberg K, Tomkowski W. Authors/Task Force Members. 2015 ESC Guidelines for the diagnosis and management of pericardial diseases: the task force for the diagnosis and management of pericardial diseases of the European Society of Cardiology (ESC) Endorsed by: The European Association for Cardio-Thoracic Surgery (EACTS). Eur Heart J. 2015;36:2921–64.
10. Imazio M, Cecchi E, Demichelis B, Chinaglia A, Ierna S, Demarie D, Ghisio A, Pomari F, Belli R, Trinchero R. Myopericarditis versus viral or idiopathic acute pericarditis. Heart. 2008;94:498–501.
11. Kytö V, Sipilä J, Rautava P. Clinical profile and influences on outcomes in patients hospitalized for acute pericarditis. Circulation. 2014;130:1601–6.
12. Imazio M, Bobbio M, Cecchi E, Demarie D, Demichelis B, Pomari F, Moratti M, Gaschino G, Giammaria M, Ghisio A, Belli R, Trinchero R. Colchicine in addition to conventional therapy for acute pericarditis: results of the COlchicine for acute PEricarditis (COPE) trial. Circulation. 2005;112:2012–6.
13. Imazio M, Brucato A, Cemin R, Ferrua S, Maggiolini S, Beqaraj F, Demarie D, Forno D, Ferro S, Maestroni S, Belli R, Trinchero R, Spodick DH, Adler Y, ICAP Investigators. A randomized trial of colchicine for acute pericarditis. N Engl J Med. 2013;369:1522–8.
14. Imazio M, Bobbio M, Cecchi E, Demarie D, Pomari F, Moratti M, Ghisio A, Belli R, Trinchero R. Colchicine as first-choice therapy for recurrent pericarditis: results of the CORE (COlchicine for REcurrent pericarditis) trial. Arch Intern Med. 2005;165:1987–91.
15. Imazio M, Brucato A, Cemin R, Ferrua S, Belli R, Maestroni S, Trinchero R, Spodick DH, Adler Y, CORP (COlchicine for Recurrent Pericarditis) Investigators. Colchicine for recurrent pericarditis (CORP): a randomized trial. Ann Intern Med. 2011;155:409–14.
16. Imazio M, Brucato A, Derosa FG, Lestuzzi C, Bombana E, Scipione F, Leuzzi S, Cecchi E, Trinchero R, Adler Y. Aetiological diagnosis in acute and recurrent pericarditis: when and how. J Cardiovasc Med (Hagerstown). 2009;10:217–30.
17. Imazio M. Pericardial involvement in systemic inflammatory diseases. Heart. 2011;97:1882–92.
18. Imazio M, Hoit BD. Post-cardiac injury syndromes. An emerging cause of pericardial diseases. Int J Cardiol. 2013;168:648–52.
19. Maisch B, Ristic A, Pankuweit S. Evaluation and management of pericardial effusion in patients with neoplastic disease. Prog Cardiovasc Dis. 2010;53:157–63.
20. Lestuzzi C, Berretta M, Tomkowski W. 2015 update on the diagnosis and management of neoplastic pericardial disease. Expert Rev Cardiovasc Ther. 2015;13:377–89.

Diagnosis: History, Physical Examination and ECG

3

3.1 History

A number of different features may be helpful in the first diagnostic evaluation to address specific pericardial syndromes and potential aetiologies to be further investigated (Table 3.1).

Symptoms of an inflammatory pericardial or myopericardial syndrome usually include chest pain, generally sharp, sudden in onset, retrosternal, pleuritic with inspiratory exacerbation (Fig. 3.1) as well as positional change: increased by lying down and attenuated during sitting and leaning forward. Pericardial pain is an example of referred pain. The cardiac general visceral sensory pain fibres follow the sympathetics back to the spinal cord. To simplify, there is a convergence of afferent signals to the same spinal cord segments from both the heart/pericardium and dermatomes of the thoracic wall and upper limb. The central nervous system does not clearly discern whether the pain is coming from the body wall or from the heart or pericardium, but it perceives the pain as coming from somewhere on the body wall, i.e. substernal pain, left arm/hand pain and jaw pain. On this basis, pericardial pain may simulate ischaemic chest pain (Fig. 3.2) [1–5].

Additional symptoms may include dyspnoea that may be caused by the exacerbation of pain with inspiration or concomitant effect of pericardial and/or pleural effusion. Non-specific symptoms include malaise, fever and cough. Fever is generally low-degree and fever >38 °C should raise the suspicion of a bacterial aetiology [1–5]. A list of potential symptoms is reported in Table 3.2.

3.2 Physical Examination

Physical findings are variable in pericardial and myopericardial diseases.

© Springer International Publishing Switzerland 2016
M. Imazio, *Myopericardial Diseases: Diagnosis and Management*,
DOI 10.1007/978-3-319-27156-9_3

Table 3.1 Features to be considered in the history of a patient with a suspected or known pericardial and myopericardial disease

	Feature
Past medical history	Previous irradiation
	Renal insufficiency with or without dialysis
	Previous infectious diseases (e.g. tuberculosis)
	Previous cardiac surgery
Recent history	Antecedent respiratory or gastrointestinal infection
	Fever (if >38 °C suggest a non-viral aetiology)
	Recent myocardial infarction
Known diseases	Systemic inflammatory diseases
	Metabolic diseases (e.g. hypothyroidism, renal insufficiency)
	Cancer (especially lung and breast cancer, lymphoma, leukaemias)[a]
Drugs	Current or recent exposure to drugs that may cause a pericardial syndrome (see Chap. 2)
	Lupus-like syndrome (procainamide, hydralazine, methyldopa, isoniazid, phenytoin)
	Hypersensitivity pericarditis with eosinophilia (e.g. penicillins)
	Other (rare), e.g. antineoplastic drugs (often associated with a cardiomyopathy, may cause a pericardiopathy), doxorubicin (Adriamycin) and daunorubicin cytosine arabinoside, 5-fluorouracil, cyclophosphamide

[a]Additional neoplasms include melanoma and cancers of contiguous anatomical structures (e.g. oesophagus)

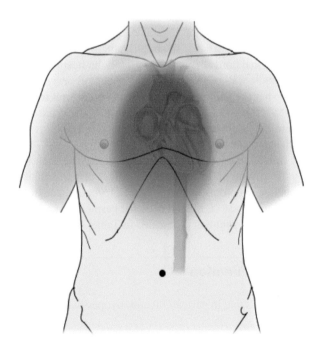

Fig. 3.1 "Pericarditic" chest pain has pleuritic features and it is usually referred as retrosternal (Reproduced from Wikipedia, Author Ian Furst)

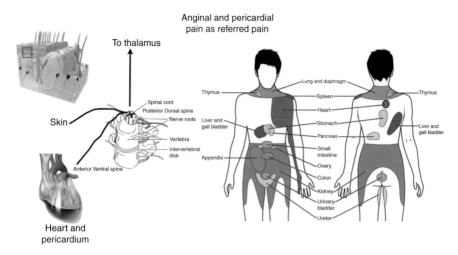

Fig. 3.2 "Pericarditic chest pain" as referred pain that may simulate "ischaemic chest pain" (Reproduced from OpenStax College, Autonomic Reflexes and Homeostasis http://cnx.org/content/m46579/1.2/)

Table 3.2 Common symptoms in pericardial and myopericardial diseases

Symptom	Pathophysiology
Chest pain (>90 % of cases)	"Pleuritic" with exacerbation with inspiration, lying down and deglutition due to increased attrition between inflamed pericardial layers
Dyspnoea	Exacerbation of pain with inspiration or concomitant effect of pericardial and/or pleural effusion and/or concomitant pleuropulmonary disease
Palpitations	Concomitant arrhythmias (e.g. supraventricular or ventricular premature beats, atrial fibrillation or flutter as most common; usually because of concomitant myocardial involvement)
Asthenia	May be related to the concomitant inflammation/infection or related to constrictive physiology developing during the pericardial disease (usually transient but may progress). May be related to cardiac tamponade
Myalgias	Usually related to the concomitant inflammation/infection and/or myopathic involvement of skeletal muscles by a potential myotropic agent
Symptoms related to compression of anatomic structures by a large effusion	Dysphagia, nausea, abdominal fullness, dyspnoea, orthopnoea
Symptoms of right heart failure	Constriction physiology

Pericardial Rubs

A patient with acute or recurrent pericarditis and myopericarditis may have a normal physical examination. In about one third of cases, a pericardial rub may be heard. A pericardial rub is supposed to be generated by increased attrition of inflamed pericardial layers. It has typically a to-and-fro character, typically with up to three components, one systolic and two diastolic (early rapid ventricular filling and atrial systole), corresponding to major changes in the size of cardiac chambers (Fig. 3.3) [1].

It resembles the sound of squeaky leather and often is described as grating, scratching or rasping. It is best heard with the patient sitting and leaning forward or in the genu-pectoral position (Fig. 3.4) since these positions enhance pericardial attrition (Fig. 3.5). The pericardial rub is a diagnostic criterion for the diagnosis of pericarditis [4–6].

Fig. 3.3 A pericardial rub may have up to three components: one systolic and two diastolic (early rapid ventricular filling and atrial systole), corresponding to major changes in the size of cardiac chambers

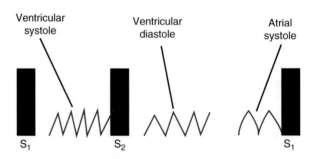

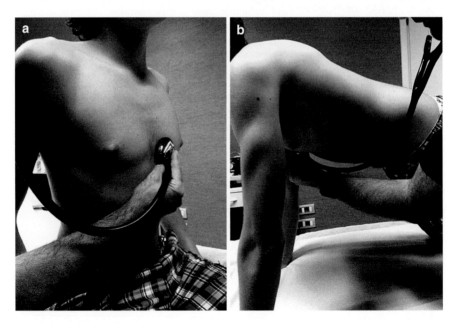

Fig. 3.4 Two positions that may enhance the chance to detect pericardial rubs: (**a**) patient is sitting and leaning forward; (**b**) genu-pectoral position with the patient lying on his/her elbows and knees

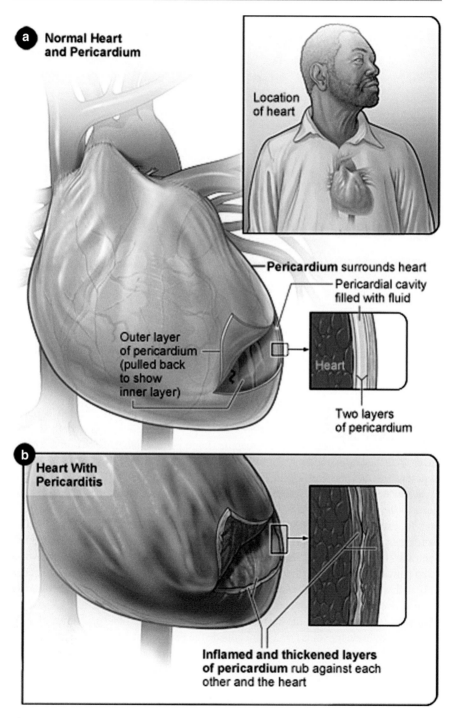

Fig. 3.5 (Panel **a**) Normal heart and pericardium. (Panel **b**) Inflamed and thickened pericardial layers rub against each other (Reproduced from Wikipedia)

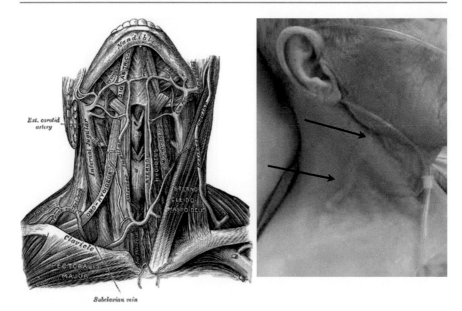

Fig. 3.6 In the setting of cardiac tamponade, two typical signs include jugular vein distension (see picture) and diminished heart sounds (Modified from Gray's Anatomy, Plate 558, and James Heilman, MD)

Physical Signs in Large Pericardial Effusions/Cardiac Tamponade

These signs include thorax dullness to percussion, distant and muffled sounds, Ewart's sign with a combination of dullness to percussion, bronchial breath sounds and aegophony at the tip of the left scapula (large pericardial effusion). In the presence of cardiac tamponade additional signs include elevated jugular vein pressure, hypotension, distant heart sound (Beck's triad) and tachycardia (Fig. 3.6) [7].

In this setting the most specific physical sign is pulsus paradoxus. *Pulsus paradoxus* is an inspiratory decrease of more than 10 mmHg of arterial systolic pressure due to exaggerated interventricular interdependence (Fig. 3.7). The inspiratory increase of venous return and right ventricle (RV) dimension is transmitted to the left ventricle (LV) by a shift of the interventricular septum (IVS) [7]. The presence of a fixed pericardial volume (either because of a large effusion or constriction) can occur only with a reduction of LV volume and thus a reduced stroke volume. Another reason for this decrease is the reduced gradient between left atrium (LA) and LV due to incomplete transmission of the inspiratory decrease of intrathoracic pressure to the LV but not the pulmonary veins (which are outside the pericardial cavity). The incomplete transmission may be due to large pericardial effusions or constrictive pericardium.

Physical Signs in Constrictive Pericarditis

In constrictive pericarditis, a rigid pericardium (which may be thickened and calcified) impairs diastolic filling, suddenly blocking the rapid ventricular filling (this sudden stop is responsible for the genesis of pericardial knock, and added

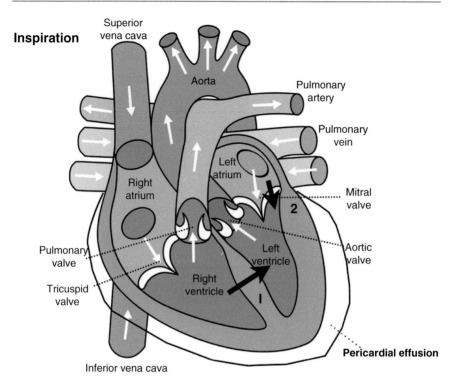

Fig. 3.7 Pulsus paradoxus. Pericardial volume and chamber volumes become fixed in the presence of large pericardial effusion/cardiac tamponade. The inspiratory decrease of systolic blood pressure is determined by (*1*) the increase venous return with increased volume of right ventricle that is responsible for a septal bounce and reduced LV volume and (*2*) decreased transmitral flow because of a reduced gradient between LA and LV (see text for additional explanation) (Modified from Wikipedia)

pathological tone). In constrictive pericarditis, the clinical picture is that of right heart failure with distended jugular veins, Kussmaul sign (paradoxical inspiratory rise in jugular venous pressure). Kussmaul sign is not specific of constrictive pericarditis since it can be seen in other heart diseases with limited right ventricular filling due to right heart failure. Additional physical signs include hepatomegaly, ascites and leg oedema [1].

3.3   Electrocardiogram

The pericardium is electrically silent; nevertheless, concomitant subepicardial involvement is common in different pericardial diseases (pericarditis, pericardial effusion, constrictive pericarditis) giving rise to electrocardiographic signs.

In *acute pericarditis*, the inflammatory involvement of the subepicardium is responsible for the appearance of *PR depression* as the earliest ECG sign, as a consequence of atrial myocardial involvement as current of injury. This ECG sign may be associated to the more commonly reported *widespread ST segment elevation* (Fig. 3.8), usually concave in shape and with the possible progression in four

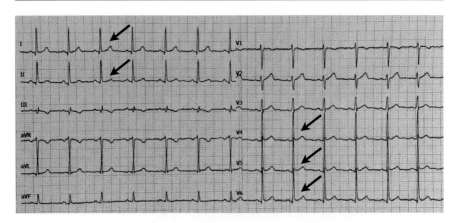

Fig. 3.8 Subacute pericarditis with mild widespread ST-segment elevation (see *black arrows*)

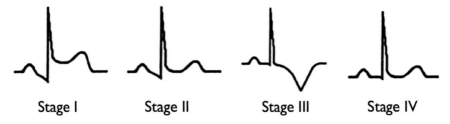

Fig. 3.9 Classical four stages of ECG evolution in acute pericarditis according to Spodick DH (see text for explanation)

classical stages (Fig. 3.9) [7–9]. The main ECG differential diagnosis is with an acute coronary syndrome and early repolarization (Table 3.3 and Fig. 3.10) [8].

The four ECG stages are the following:

Stage I: Acute phase: PR depression and/or widespread ST segment elevation
Stage II: ST segment on the isoelectric line without T wave inversion
Stage III: T wave inversion
Stage IV: Normalization

Such evolution may be affected by prompt medical therapy and the ECG presentation is affected by the presentation time. Patients with an acute presentation will show a widespread ST segment elevation; on the contrary, chronic cases may only display T wave inversion. A patient with a prompt remission may have a normal ECG. In any case widespread ST-segment elevation is a diagnostic criterion for pericarditis and it is reported in about 60 % of patients with acute pericarditis and in >2 of 3 of those with myopericarditis. The classical ECG evolution of pericarditis is reported in no more than 50 % of cases [1].

Table 3.3 ECG differential diagnosis: acute pericarditis vs. ST-segment elevation myocardial infarction (STEMI)

ECG feature	Acute pericarditis	Early repolarization	STEMI
PR depression	Possible	No	No
ST elevation	Concave up	Concave up	Usually convex
Localization of ST elevation	Widespread	Usually precordial, inferior leads	Localized
Reciprocal ST changes	No	No	Common
T wave inversion	Yes but after ST-segment normalization	No	Yes before ST-segment normalization
ST/T ratio in lead V6	>0.25	<0.25	Variable
Presence of Q waves	No	No	Possible
QT prolongation	No	No	Possible

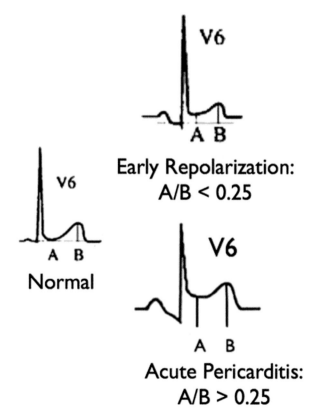

Fig. 3.10 The height of the J point can be used to differentiate early repolarization from acute pericarditis. If A/B is <0.25, early repolarization is diagnosed

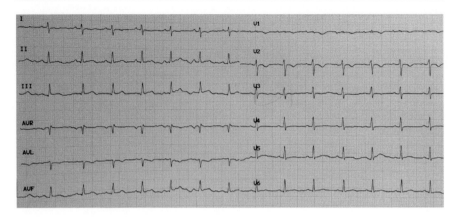

Fig. 3.11 Low QRS voltages and aspecific ST/T changes in a chronic large idiopathic pericardial effusion (see text for explanation)

Additional ECG changes are rather non-specific and can be detected in the presence of large pericardial effusions and cardiac tamponade: *low QRS voltages* and *electrical alternans* [7].

Low QRS voltages (Fig. 3.11) on the ECG is defined as a QRS amplitude of <0.5 mV (or 5 mm) in the limb leads and/or <1 mV (or 10 mm) in the precordial leads. It is a non-sensitive, non-specific sign that occurs in large pericardial effusion/cardiac tamponade due to reduced transmission of ECG voltages on the body surface. Alternative causes to be considered include hypothyroidism, chronic obstructive pulmonary diseases, infiltrative heart diseases (e.g. amyloidosis), advanced heart failure and chronic ischaemic heart disease, pleural effusion, pneumothorax and obesity. *Non-specific repolarization abnormalities* (ST segment/T waves) can be also recorded in patients with large pericardial effusion/cardiac tamponade, chronic pericarditis and constrictive pericarditis [1, 7].

Electrical alternans is a beat-to-beat alternation of QRS complex amplitude and it is seen in cardiac tamponade and severe pericardial effusions. It is thought to be related to changes in the ventricular electrical axis due a swinging heart into the pericardial fluid (Figs. 3.8 and 3.12) [1, 7].

Cardiac arrhythmias are rare in pericardial diseases in the absence of concomitant structural heart diseases or myocardial involvement, such as in myopericarditis/perimyocarditis. In recent prospective studies on consecutive patients with acute pericarditis, the most common arrhythmias were extrasystoles followed by atrial fibrillation and flutter (AF/f). AF/f was reported in 4–5 % of cases, especially in older patients and with pericardial effusion. AF/f usually developed within 24 h of pericarditis and lasted >24 h only in 25 % and spontaneously converted in about 75 % of patients. Underlying structural heart disease was present in 15–20 % of cases. In a 30-month follow-up, patients with history AF/f at the initial episode had a higher rate of arrhythmia recurrence (one third recurred), mostly (75 %) within 3 months [10].

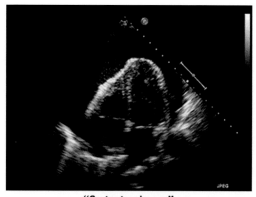

"Swinging heart"

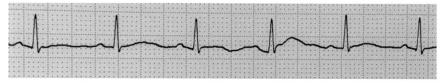

Electrical alternans= beat to beat alternation of QRS
complex amplitude

Fig. 3.12 Electrical alternans (see explanation in text)

The occurrence of AF/f in acute pericarditis identifies a predisposed population to AF/f with a high recurrence risk: in these patients, pericarditis is an arrhythmic trigger and oral anticoagulation should be seriously considered according to guideline recommendation.

Key Points
- A number of different features may be helpful in the first diagnostic evaluation to address a specific pericardial syndrome and potential aetiologies to be further investigated.
- History should be based on past and recent medical history, known diseases that may be cause of pericardial disease and drugs.
- Symptoms of pericardial diseases are varied: the most common is chest pain that is generally sharp, sudden in onset, retrosternal, pleuritic with inspiratory exacerbation and postural changes.
- Physical signs are variable according to the pericardial syndrome and include pericardial rubs (pericarditis), elevated jugular vein pressure, hypotension, muffled heart sound, pulsus paradoxus (cardiac tamponade) and signs of right heart failure in case of constrictive pericarditis.

- The pericardium is electrically silent; nevertheless, concomitant subepicardial involvement is common in different pericardial diseases (pericarditis, pericardial effusion, constrictive pericarditis) giving rise to electrocardiographic signs.
- Additional ECG signs in large pericardial effusions and cardiac tamponade include low QRS voltages and electrical alternans.
- Cardiac arrhythmias are rare in pericardial diseases in the absence of concomitant structural heart diseases or myocardial involvement, such as in myopericarditis/perimyocarditis.

References

1. Imazio M, Spodick DH, Brucato A, Trinchero R, Markel G, Adler Y. Diagnostic issues in the clinical management of pericarditis. Int J Clin Pract. 2010;64:1384–92.
2. Imazio M, Spodick DH, Brucato A, Trinchero R, Adler Y. Controversial issues in the management of pericardial diseases. Circulation. 2010;121:916–28.
3. Imazio M. Contemporary management of pericardial diseases. Curr Opin Cardiol. 2012;27:308–17.
4. LeWinter MM. Clinical practice. Acute pericarditis. N Engl J Med. 2014;371:2410–6.
5. Imazio M, Gaita F. Diagnosis and treatment of pericarditis. Heart. 2015;101:1159–68.
6. Ariyarajah V, Spodick DH. Acute pericarditis: diagnostic cues and common electrocardiographic manifestations. Cardiol Rev. 2007;15:24–30.
7. Roy CL, Minor MA, Brookhart MA, Choudhry NK. Does this patient with a pericardial effusion have cardiac tamponade? JAMA. 2007;297:1810–8.
8. Pollak P, Brady W. Electrocardiographic patterns mimicking ST segment elevation myocardial infarction. Cardiol Clin. 2012;30:601–15.
9. Punja M, Mark DG, McCoy JV, Javan R, Pines JM, Brady W. Electrocardiographic manifestations of cardiac infectious-inflammatory disorders. Am J Emerg Med. 2010;28:364–77.
10. Imazio M, Lazaros G, Picardi E, Vasileiou P, Orlando F, Carraro M, Tsiachris D, Vlachopoulos C, Georgiopoulos G, Tousoulis D, Belli R, Gaita F. Incidence and prognostic significance of new onset atrial fibrillation/flutter in acute pericarditis. Heart. 2015;101:1463–7.

Multimodality Imaging of Pericardial/ Myopericardial Diseases

4

4.1 Introduction

A modern approach of patients with a suspected pericardial and myopericardial diseases includes the availability of multimodality imaging to assess more complex cases and perform an appropriate aetiological search as well as assessment of diagnostic and prognostic features that affect the clinical management.

The basic clinical evaluation has been reviewed in the previous chapter and should include echocardiography as a first-level, mandatory diagnostic and follow-up study of patients.

Previous and current European guidelines, as well as Spanish, Brazilian guidelines on the management of pericardial diseases and American and European consensus documents gave a strong recommendation to perform echocardiography in all patients with a suspicion of pericardial diseases (Class I indication, Level of Evidence C) (Table 4.1) [1–6].

More common second-level imaging techniques include computed tomography (CT) and cardiac magnetic resonance (CMR).

Before briefly reviewing the indications, relative strengths and weaknesses of each main imaging technique, it is important not to forget the role of chest x-ray.

4.2 Chest X-Ray

Chest x-ray is a first-level imaging modality in patients with a suspected pericarditis or pericardial effusion in order to detect the presence of a cardiomegaly (may suggest a pericardial effusion), pericardial calcifications (chronic and constrictive pericarditis) and/or concomitant pleuropulmonary disease as first screening (e.g. pleural effusion, pneumonia, tuberculosis, lung cancer and hilar and mediastinal enlargement) (Fig. 4.1).

In a patient with pericarditis and without significant structural heart diseases, the chest x-ray may be absolutely normal (Fig. 4.2). A pericardial effusion is able to

© Springer International Publishing Switzerland 2016   27
M. Imazio, *Myopericardial Diseases: Diagnosis and Management*,
DOI 10.1007/978-3-319-27156-9_4

Table 4.1   Classes of recommendations and levels of evidence in European guidelines

Classes	Definition	Clinical indication
I	Evidence and/or general agreement in favour	It is recommended
II	Conflicting evidence	To be considered
III	Evidence and/or general agreement is against it	It is not recommended

Level of Evidence (*LOE*): (a) data derived from multiple randomized controlled trials (RCTs) or meta-analyses; (b) data derived from a single RCT or large non-randomized studies; (c) experts consensus, small prospective studies, retrospectives studies and registries

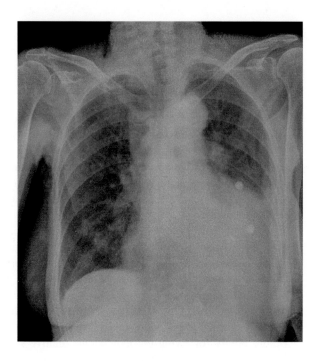

Fig. 4.1   A 78-year-old woman with pleuropericarditis and pneumonia. Cardiomegaly due to pericardial effusion and concomitant left pleural effusion

increase the size of the cardiac silhouette only if >300 mL, and cardiac silhouette may assume a "bottle" shape in the presence of large pericardial effusions, especially when chronic and slowly accumulating (Fig. 4.3) [2].

4.3   Echocardiography

Transthoracic echocardiography is the first-line imaging test in patients with suspected pericardial disease (Class I indication, LOE C) [2]. One of the first applications of echocardiography was the detection of pericardial effusion. Even nowadays, echocardiography offers the simplest and cheapest diagnostic option to detect the presence of pericardial effusion, providing a semiquantitative assessment of the

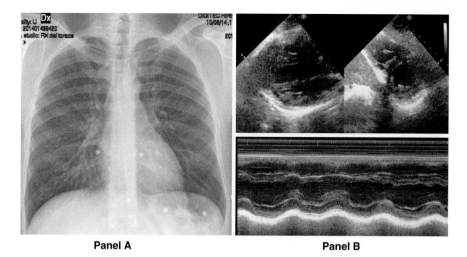

Panel A   **Panel B**

Fig. 4.2 A patient with acute pericarditis and a normal chest-x-ray (panel **a**). Non-specific pericardial brightness on echocardiography (panel **b**)

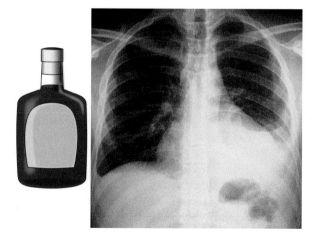

Fig. 4.3 A pericardial effusion of >300 mL is responsible for an enlargement of cardiac silhouette that can be detected on chest x-ray

size, that can be easily performed even at bedside and in urgent/emergency settings.

In clinical practice, the size of pericardial effusion on M-mode, 2D echocardiography is qualitatively assessed by the end-diastolic distance of the echo-free space between the epicardium and parietal pericardium: small (<10 mm), moderate (10–20 mm) and large (>20 mm) (Fig. 4.4) [2]. Pericardial fluid accumulates following available spaces and gravity forces. On the left lateral decubitus, the fluid starts accumulating posteriorly (mild effusions), and then after the complete filling of the

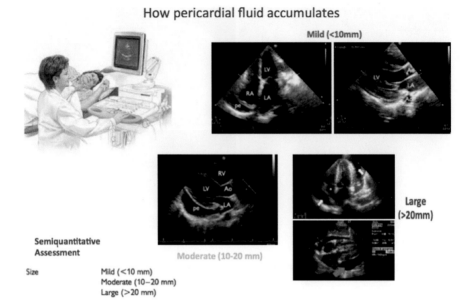

Fig. 4.4 Semiquantitative assessment of pericardial effusion (see text for explanation)

posterior space, pericardial effusion becomes circumferential. On this basis, an iso-lated anterior pericardial echo-free space should be considered as evidence of increased epicardial fat instead of pericardial fluid, especially in the absence of previous cardiac surgery, trauma or pericarditis with or without interventional pro-cedures. CT and CMR may provide better tissue characterization of the echo-free space (Fig. 4.5).

Additional contributes of echocardiography include follow-up studies for peri-cardial effusions, assessment of cardiac tamponade, constrictive features, evalua-tion of left and right ventricular function and kinesis, as well as concomitant structural heart diseases. A detailed discussion on echocardiographic features of cardiac tamponade and constrictive pericarditis will be reviewed in the specific chapter on these pericardial syndromes. On echocardiography, a concomitant pleu-ral effusion can be detected. Left pleural effusion can be differentiated from pericar-dial effusion since pleural effusion is posterior to the thoracic descending aorta (Fig. 4.6).

4.4   Computed Tomography (CT)

The normal pericardium is visible as a thin curvilinear structure surrounded by the hypodense mediastinal and epicardial fat and has a thickness ranging between 0.7 and 2.0 mm. The pericardial sinuses and their respective recesses are well visible on computed tomography (CT).

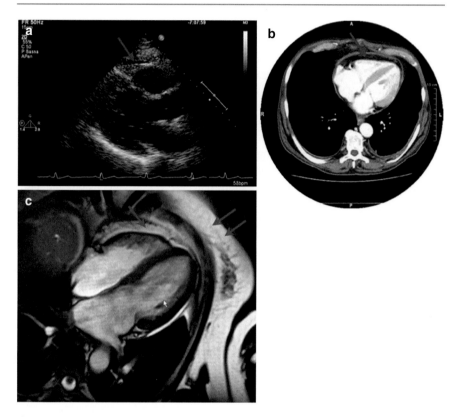

Fig. 4.5 Multimodality imaging of epicardial fat: an echo-free space on echocardiography (panel **a**) that is better characterized on CT (panel **b**) and especially on CMR (panel **c**). *Single red arrows* indicating epicardial fat, while *double arrows* indicate subcutaneous fat (note the same appearance of epicardial fat on CMR)

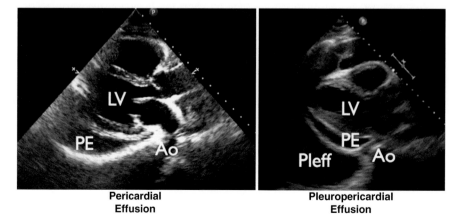

Fig. 4.6 Left pleural effusion (*Pleff*) lies posteriorly to thoracic descending aorta (*Ao*), while pericardial effusion (*PE*) is located anteriorly. *LV* Left Ventricle

CT is a second-level complementary imaging modality that is especially useful for the study of pericardial calcifications as well as concomitant pleuropulmonary diseases. In addition, CT may be helpful to provide some tissue characterization of pericardial fluid. Attenuation values of pericardial fluid (HU) yield information with regard to nature of fluid: low attenuation values (e.g. 0–20 HU) indicate a simple effusion and a transudate, intermediate values (e.g. 20–60 HU) are suggestive of a proteinaceous, exudative effusions, while high attenuation values (>60 HU) suggest haemorrhage [7–10].

CT is the most accurate technique to image calcified tissue, and it is especially helpful to depict the extension of calcifications allowing a better surgical plan for pericardiectomy. Nowadays modern multi-detector CT scanners combine both acquisition speed and high contrast and spatial resolution providing excellent anatomical details. Low-radiation cardiac CT is feasible using prospective electrocardiographic triggering. In clinical practice, CT provides limited contribution to the functional study of the heart and pericardium [2, 10]. Intravenous administration of iodinated contrast material is able to detect pericardial inflammation since the inflamed pericardium is enhanced after contrast injection.

Additional contribution of CT studies includes the evaluation and diagnosis of pericardial masses and cysts and the congenital partial or complete absence of the pericardium.

4.5   Cardiac Magnetic Resonance (CMR)

Cardiac magnetic resonance (CMR) is another second-level imaging technique for the study of pericardial and myopericardial diseases [2].

Similar to CT, the normal pericardium appears as a thin hypointense ("dark") curvilinear structure surrounded by hyperintense ("bright") mediastinal and epicardial fat on T1-weighted imaging. Normal pericardial thickness is less than 2 mm (Fig. 4.7).

The inflamed pericardium can be seen on short tau inversion-recovery (STIR) T2-weighted images providing evidence of pericardial oedema, and it also shows late gadolinium enhancement providing evidence of organizing pericarditis and fibrosis (Fig. 4.8).

Additional contribution of CMR include:

1. Characterization of pericardial fluid
2. Assessment of concomitant constrictive physiology (pericardial thickening, adhesions on tagging, septal bounce on cine real-time images)
3. Assessment of concomitant myocarditis
4. Study of pericardial masses and cysts
5. Study of congenital abnormalities of the pericardium
6. Evaluation of concomitant heart and pleuropulmonary diseases

The main limitation of CMR is the limited availability in many clinical settings, the costs, the need of breath-holding and regular cardiac rhythms to achieve better image quality [11–13].

Fig. 4.7 The normal pericardium (*red arrows*) on T1-weighted CMR imaging (see text for explanation)

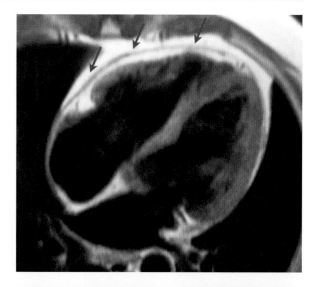

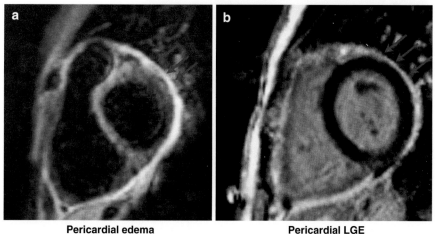

Pericardial edema   Pericardial LGE

Fig. 4.8 Patient with acute pericarditis on CMR study: evidence of pericardial oedema (panel **a**: *red arrows*) plus late gadolinium enhancement (*LGE*: *red arrows*; panel **b**)

4.6 Nuclear Medicine

Nuclear medicine imaging techniques have specific indication in selected cases to assess the metabolic activity of the pericardium, especially in suspected neoplastic pericardial disease or infectious pericarditis, such as tuberculous pericarditis. PET alone or preferably in combination with CT (PET/CT) is commonly utilized for this diagnostic application. Pericardial uptake of (18)F-fluorodeoxyglucose (FDG) tracer in patients with solid cancers and lymphoma is indicative of malignant pericardial involvement (Fig. 4.9). The clinical application of this technique ranges from diagnosis to staging and assessment of therapeutic response [14–17].

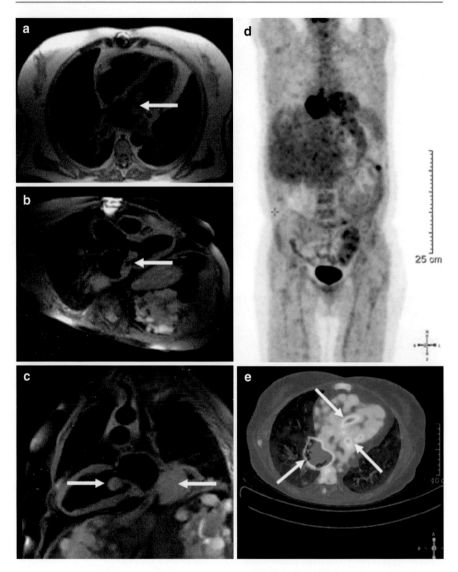

Fig. 4.9 53-year-old female with not-otherwise-specified sarcoma (NOS, *arrows*) at the pericardium involving the lung and mitral valve in T1-weighted 4-chamber (**a**, T2-weighted single-slice turbo spin-echo sequence without fat saturation), 3-chamber (**b**) and fat-saturated and contrast-enhanced long-axis (**c**) views (both: T2-weighted single-slice turbo spin-echo sequence with fat saturation). PET imaging shows the moderate cardiac (around the mitral valve) and the marked pulmonary FDG uptake (**d**). PET images are superimposed to CT findings (**e**). (Reproduced with permission from [14])

4.7   Multimodality Imaging

In more complex cases, the integration of second-level imaging techniques is essential for the diagnosis (Fig. 4.10). Each technique has its own indications, strengths and weaknesses (Table 4.2) [8, 9].

To summarize, echocardiography remains the first-level essential imaging testing with a wide availability, limited costs and opportunity to be performed in most settings, including bedside, urgent and emerging settings. Echocardiography is however weak for the assessment of pericardial thickening, calcifications, inflammation as well as concomitant pleuropulmonary diseases.

CT is the second-level imaging that offers the best opportunity to study pericardial calcifications and offers also the opportunity to study pericardial inflammation, masses, effusions and concomitant pleuropulmonary diseases. It is relatively widely available and has limited costs but requires breath-holding, iodinated contrast and the use of ionizing radiation [10].

CMR is the second-level imaging modality of choice for the study of pericardial and myocardial inflammation as well as tissue characterization and functional studies in patients with a suspicion of constrictive physiology [18, 19]. Unfortunately it is not widely available; it is expensive and time consuming and can be performed only in stable patients. Both CT and CMR techniques may be seriously affected by cardiac arrhythmias [20, 21].

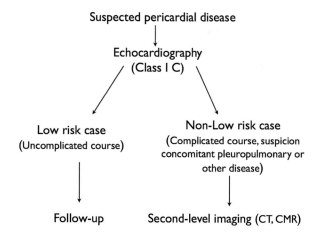

Fig. 4.10 Indications for echocardiography and second-level imaging techniques in patients with suspected pericardial diseases

Table 4.2 Indications, strengths and weaknesses of imaging techniques for pericardial and myopericardial diseases

	Echocardiography	CT	CMR
Indications	First-level assessment and follow-up study for pericardial diseases	Second-level imaging technique (best for assessment of calcifications)	Second-level imaging technique (best for tissue characterization and assessment of inflammation)
Main strengths	Widely available, cheap, Use in urgent/ emergency settings and bedside Safe and repeatable	Better anatomic study Evaluation of concomitant pleuropulmonary diseases Evaluation of calcifications	Better anatomic study Evaluation of concomitant pleuropulmonary diseases Assessment of pericardial and myocardial inflammation
Main weaknesses	Limited windows Operator dependent Limited tissue characterization Poor quality imaging	Use of ionizing radiation Use of iodinated contrast Limited functional study Difficult in cardiac arrhythmias Need for breath-hold Only stable patients	Time consuming Limited availability High costs Not good for pericardial calcifications Difficult in cardiac arrhythmias Need for breath-hold Only stable patients

Key Points
- Echocardiography is the first choice imaging modality in any patients with a clinical suspicion of pericardial disease.
- Multimodality imaging should be considered in complicated cases, when echocardiography is not conclusive or a concomitant disease is suspected (e.g. cancer, tuberculosis).
- CT and CMR are second-level imaging modalities.
- CT is especially useful for the study of pericardial thickening and calcifications.
- CMR is especially useful for the characterization of pericardial effusions and masses and to depict pericardial and myocardial inflammation.
- Access to multimodality imaging is necessary for the diagnosis, stratification and management of more complex cases with pericardial diseases.

References

1. Maisch B, Seferović PM, Ristić AD, Erbel R, Rienmüller R, Adler Y, Tomkowski WZ, Thiene G, Yacoub MH, Task Force on the Diagnosis and Management of Pericardial Diseases of the European Society of Cardiology. Guidelines on the diagnosis and management of pericardial

diseases executive summary; the task force on the diagnosis and management of pericardial diseases of the European society of cardiology. Eur Heart J. 2004;25:587–610.

2. Authors/Task Force Members, Adler Y, Charron P, Imazio M, Badano L, Barón-Esquivias G, Bogaert J, Brucato A, Gueret P, Klingel K, Lionis C, Maisch B, Mayosi B, Pavie A, Ristić AD, Sabaté Tenas M, Seferovic P, Swedberg K, Tomkowski W. 2015 ESC guidelines for the diagnosis and management of pericardial diseases: the task force for the diagnosis and management of pericardial diseases of the European Society of Cardiology (ESC)endorsed by: the European Association for Cardio-Thoracic Surgery (EACTS). Eur Heart J. 2015;36:2921–64.

3. Sagristá Sauleda J, Almenar Bonet L, Angel Ferrer J, Bardají Ruiz A, Bosch Genover X, Guindo Soldevila J, Mercé Klein J, Permanyer Miralda C, Tello de Meneses Becerra R. [The clinical practice guidelines of the Sociedad Española de Cardiología on pericardial pathology]. Rev Esp Cardiol. 2000;53:394–412.

4. Montera MW, Mesquita ET, Colafranceschi AS, Oliveira Jr Jr AC, Rabischoffsky A, Ianni BM, Rochitte CE, Mady C, Mesquita CT, Azevedo CF, Bocchi EA, Saad EB, Braga FG, Fernandes F, Ramires FJ, Bacal F, Feitosa GS, Figueira HR, Souza Neto JD, Moura LA, Campos LA, Bittencourt MI, Barbosa Mde M, Moreira Mda C, Higuchi Mde L, Schwartzmann P, Rocha RM, Pereira SB, Mangini S, Martins SM, Bordignon S, Salles VA, Sociedade Brasileira de Cardiologia. I Brazilian guidelines on myocarditis and pericarditis. Arq Bras Cardiol. 2013;100(4 Suppl 1):1–36.

5. Klein AL, Abbara S, Agler DA, Appleton CP, Asher CR, Hoit B, Hung J, Garcia MJ, Kronzon I, Oh JK, Rodriguez ER, Schaff HV, Schoenhagen P, Tan CD, White RD. American Society of Echocardiography clinical recommendations for multimodality cardiovascular imaging of patients with pericardial disease: endorsed by the Society for Cardiovascular Magnetic Resonance and Society of Cardiovascular Computed Tomography. J Am Soc Echocardiogr. 2013;26:965–1012.

6. Cosyns B, Plein S, Nihoyanopoulos P, Smiseth O, Achenbach S, Andrade MJ, Pepi M, Ristic A, Imazio M, Paelinck B, Lancellotti P, European Association of Cardiovascular Imaging (EACVI), European Society of Cardiology Working Group (ESC WG) on Myocardial and Pericardial Diseases. European Association of Cardiovascular Imaging (EACVI) position paper: multimodality imaging in pericardial disease. Eur Heart J Cardiovasc Imaging. 2015;16:12–31.

7. Seferović PM, Ristić AD, Maksimović R, Simeunović DS, Milinković I, Seferović Mitrović JP, Kanjuh V, Pankuweit S, Maisch B. Pericardial syndromes: an update after the ESC guidelines 2004. Heart Fail Rev. 2013;18:255–66.

8. Verhaert D, Gabriel RS, Johnston D, Lytle BW, Desai MY, Klein AL. The role of multimodality imaging in the management of pericardial disease. Circ Cardiovasc Imaging. 2010;3:333–43.

9. Yared K, Baggish AL, Picard MH, Hoffmann U, Hung J. Multimodality imaging of pericardial disease. J Am Coll Cardiol Img. 2010;3:650–60.

10. Bogaert J, Francone M. Pericardial disease: value of CT and MR imaging. Radiology. 2013;267:340–56.

11. Frank H, Globits S. Magnetic resonance imaging evaluation of myocardial and pericardial disease. J Magn Reson Imaging. 1999;10:617–26.

12. Bogaert J, Francone M. Cardiovascular magnetic resonance in pericardial diseases. J Cardiovasc Magn Reson. 2009;11:14.

13. Misselt AJ, Harris SR, Glockner J, Feng D, Syed IS, Araoz PA. MR imaging of the pericardium. Magn Reson Imaging Clin N Am. 2008;16:185–99.

14. Alter P, Figiel JH, Rupp TP, Bachmann GF, Maisch B, Rominger MB. MR, CT, and PET imaging in pericardial disease. Heart Fail Rev. 2013;18:289–306.

15. Dawson D, Rubens M, Mohiaddin R. Contemporary imaging of the pericardium. J Am Coll Cardiol Img. 2011;4:680–4.

16. Lobert P, Brown RK, Dvorak RA, Corbett JR, Kazerooni EA, Wong KK. Spectrum of physiological and pathological cardiac and pericardial uptake of FDG in oncology PET-CT. Clin Radiol. 2013;68:e59–71.

17. James OG, Christensen JD, Wong T, Borges-Neto S, Koweek LM. Utility of FDG PET/CT in inflammatory cardiovascular disease. Radiographics. 2011;31:1271–86.
18. Alraies MC, AlJaroudi W, Yarmohammadi H, Yingchoncharoen T, Schuster A, Senapati A, Tariq M, Kwon D, Griffin BP, Klein AL. Usefulness of cardiac magnetic resonance-guided management in patients with recurrent pericarditis. Am J Cardiol. 2015;115:542–7.
19. Feng D, Glockner J, Kim K, Martinez M, Syed IS, Araoz P, Breen J, Espinosa RE, Sundt T, Schaff HV, Oh JK. Cardiac magnetic resonance imaging pericardial late gadolinium enhancement and elevated inflammatory markers can predict the reversibility of constrictive pericarditis after antiinflammatory medical therapy: a pilot study. Circulation. 2011;124:1830–7.
20. Imazio M. Contemporary management of pericardial diseases. Curr Opin Cardiol. 2012;27:308–17.
21. Imazio M, Gaita F. Diagnosis and treatment of pericardis. Heart. 2015;101(14):1159–68.

Cardiac Catheterization and Interventional Techniques

5

5.1 Cardiac Catheterization

Historically, cardiac catheterization has been a mainstay for the diagnosis of cardiac tamponade, constrictive pericarditis and cardiac tamponade. Nowadays, the widespread use of alternative non-invasive diagnostic techniques has seriously limited the role of cardiac catheterization to complex cases, where there are conflicting data from clinical evaluation and non-invasive imaging for constrictive pericarditis or restrictive cardiomyopathy or emergency/urgent settings where cardiac tamponade develops during invasive procedures (e.g. coronary angioplasty, pacemaker implantation or arrhythmias ablation) and requires immediate diagnosis and treatment [1–4].

Cardiac Tamponade

It is only rarely diagnosed by cardiac haemodymamics. Cardiac tamponade develops when cardiac filling is impaired by intrapericardial pressure exceeding intracardiac pressures, resulting in impaired ventricular filling during the entire diastolic time.

The classical haemodynamic picture includes arterial hypotension, pulsus paradoxus (see Chap. 3) and atrial pressure that is typically elevated, with prominent x descents and blunted or absent y descents (Fig. 5.1). Blunted or absent y descent is secondary to diastolic equalization of pressures in the right atrium and right ventricle and lack of effective flow across the tricuspid valve in early ventricular diastole [3].

Constrictive Pericarditis

In constrictive pericarditis, a rigid pericardium that may be thickened or not thickened fixes the total volume of cardiac chambers, dissociates the intrathoracic pressures from intracardiac pressures and impairs diastolic filling in mid and late diastole (Fig. 5.2) [1, 3].

© Springer International Publishing Switzerland 2016
M. Imazio, *Myopericardial Diseases: Diagnosis and Management*,
DOI 10.1007/978-3-319-27156-9_5

Fig. 5.1 Hemodynamic tracing of atrial pressure in cardiac tamponade showing blunted or absent y descent (panel A) and normal conditions (panel B). *RA* Right Atrium, * is used to underline the changes

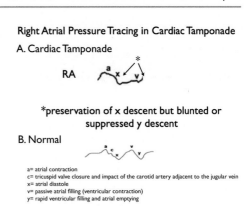

Right Atrial Pressure Tracing in Cardiac Tamponade

A. Cardiac Tamponade

RA

*preservation of x descent but blunted or suppressed y descent

B. Normal

a= atrial contraction
c= tricuspid valve closure and impact of the carotid artery adjacent to the jugular vein
x= atrial diastole
v= passive atrial filling (ventricular contraction)
y= rapid ventricular filling and atrial emptying

Fig. 5.2 Pathophysiology of constrictive pericarditis. The diastolic ventricular filling is impaired in mid- and late diastole; thus, the early diastolic filling is quick and suddenly halted by the rigid pericardium in mid-diastole

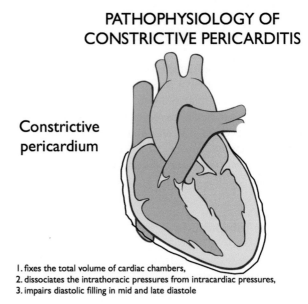

PATHOPHYSIOLOGY OF CONSTRICTIVE PERICARDITIS

Constrictive pericardium

1. fixes the total volume of cardiac chambers,
2. dissociates the intrathoracic pressures from intracardiac pressures,
3. impairs diastolic filling in mid and late diastole

The main differential diagnosis is with restrictive cardiomyopathy (rCMP). In this pathological condition, diastolic filling is impaired because of a disease of the myocardium and not the external envelope; thus, diastolic dysfunction is present and primarily affects the left ventricle, and high filling pressures are recorded in all cardiac chambers; moreover there is no dissociation of intrathoracic pressures and intracardiac pressures.

The *classical haemodynamic criteria* for the differentiation of rCMP from constrictive pericarditis include [1, 3, 4]:

1. LV end-diastolic pressure (LVEDP) exceeds RV end-diastolic pressure (RVEDP) by 5 mmHg or more.
2. In RV, the RVEDP is less than 1/3 of systolic pressure.
3. Pulmonary artery systolic pressure is greater than 50 mmHg.

In addition in constrictive pericarditis, cardiac catheterization shows:

1. Dip and plateau pattern of ventricular pressure curves (Fig. 5.3) during early diastole and rapid x and y descents of atrial pressures curves (as can be seen in rCMP)
2. Dissociation of intracavitary and intrathoracic pressures with inspiratory decrease of LV pressure and increase of RV pressure with enhancement of ventricular interdependence and discordant changes in LV and RV pressures during respiration (only in constrictive pericarditis)

This respiratory reciprocal changes of ventricular pressures can be quantified using a systolic area index (SAI) that has been proposed by the Mayo Clinic investigators (Fig. 5.4) [5].

5.2   Pericardiocentesis

Pericardiocentesis is the interventional technique to drain pericardial fluid by a percutaneous route. It has been first developed as blinded or ECG-guided technique by a subxiphoid approach (Fig. 5.5). Nowadays, due to the high possible complication risk, pericardiocentesis should be no more blinded or ECG guided, and essentially it can be performed by echocardiographic guidance to assess the place where the size of pericardial effusion is largest and closest to the thoracic surface or by

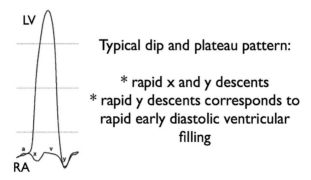

Fig. 5.3 Dip and plateau pattern of constrictive pericarditis (see text for explanation)

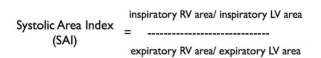

Fig. 5.4 Systolic area index (*SAI*). A SAI ratio >1.1 has 97 % sensitivity and 100 % predictive accuracy to identify patients with constrictive pericarditis (this ratio has been validated in a study with surgically proven constrictive pericarditis)

Pericardiocentesis
Classical Subxiphoid Approach

Needle is inserted
between xiphoid process
and costal margin with a
30 to 45° angle towards
the left mid-clavicle

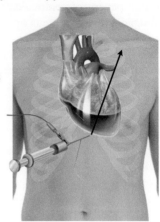

Fig. 5.5 Classical pericardiocentesis by a subxiphoid approach and ECG monitoring that should be no more performed. Guidance should be provided by echocardiography (most settings) or fluoroscopy

fluoroscopic guidance especially when cardiac tamponade occurs in the cath lab as complication of a diagnostic or therapeutic interventional technique [4, 6].

Main indications for pericardiocentesis include:

1. Cardiac tamponade (therapeutic and diagnostic pericardiocentesis)
2. Moderate to large, symptomatic pericardial effusion not responding to medical therapy (therapeutic and diagnostic pericardiocentesis)
3. Suspicion of bacterial or neoplastic aetiology of pericardial effusion (diagnostic pericardiocentesis), since the definite diagnosis would require the isolation of the aetiological agent in pericardial fluid (or tissue)

The standard technique for pericardiocentesis is guided by echocardiography or fluoroscopy under local anaesthesia. Blind procedures must be not be used to avoid the risk of laceration of the heart or other organs, except in very rare situations that are immediately life threatening. An experienced operator and staff should perform pericardiocentesis in a facility equipped for radiographic, echocardiographic, haemodynamic and ECG monitoring [6, 7].

For *echo-guided pericardiocentesis*, the entry site is defined by echocardiography that allows identifying the point of the body surface where the pericardial fluid collection is maximal and closest to the thorax. The use of specific devices may allow monitoring the procedure during all the time (*echo-monitored pericardiocentesis*).

For *fluoroscopic-guided pericardiocentesis*, the entry site is subxiphoid, and the lateral angiographic view provides the best visualization of the puncturing needle and its relation to the diaphragm and the pericardium.

To verify the position of the needle or if haemorrhagic fluid is aspirated, it is possible to inject agitated saline during the echo-guided procedure or a few millilitres of contrast medium under fluoroscopic control to verify the correct position of the needle.

Regardless the guidance, the needle is inserted at the entry site and advanced with gentle aspiration into the pericardial space till fluid is obtained. Then a soft J-tip guidewire is then introduced and exchanged for a multi-hole pigtail catheter, through which the evacuation of the fluid is done. It is generally recommended not to evacuate large amount of fluid in order to prevent a rare, but potentially fatal complication of fast pericardiocentesis, named the *cardiac decompression syndrome* and manifested by paradoxical hemodynamic deterioration, ventricular dysfunction and pulmonary oedema after pericardiocentesis (Fig. 5.6). In order to prevent the complication, it is appropriate to drain pericardial fluid till resolution of the cardiac tamponade (may be assessed by echocardiography or hemodynamic pressures recording) and in any case no more than 500 mL and then to keep pericardial drainage till a daily return <25–30 mL [8].

The pericardial fluid is then removed using a vacuum bottle or manual techniques to promote the apposition of pericardial layers. Nevertheless, it is thought that in order to prevent reaccumulation of pericardial fluid, it is more important the irritating effect of the drainage tube that promote local inflammation with adhesion of pericardial layers.

The drainage should be aspirated every 4–6 h and flushed with heparinized saline in order to realize full drainage of pericardial fluid.

Pericardiocentesis should be performed by experienced operators and carries a variable risk of complications from 4 to 10 % depending on the type of monitoring,

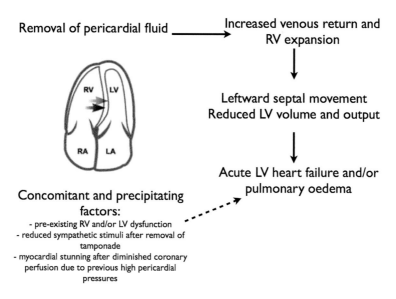

Fig. 5.6 The cardiac decompression syndrome following pericardiocentesis

skills of the operator and setting (emergency vs. urgent vs. elective). Most common complications include arrhythmias, coronary artery or cardiac chamber puncture, haemothorax, pneumothorax, pneumopericardium and hepatic injury.

Pericardiocentesis is a more dangerous procedure when pericardial fluid is not free and in lateral or posterior located or <10 mm. In these cases a surgical approach might be safer depending on local expertise and availability [9, 10].

5.3   Pericardioscopy, Pericardial Biopsy and Intrapericardial Therapies

In specialized, tertiary referral centres, endoscopic study of the pericardium may be possible through subxiphoid percutaneous approach. This technique is known as pericardioscopy, and it is usually performed by a flexible bronchoscopy endoscopic tube [9].

It can allow direct visualization of the pericardial sac with its epicardial and pericardial layers and targeted biopsies from epicardial and pericardial layers, avoiding epicardial vessels and increasing the probability of getting disease-specific results.

Experience of this technique is quite demanding, and it is possible to do it only in a limited number of experienced tertiary referral centres (e.g. Marburg, Germany or Belgrade, Serbia) [9].

Access to pericardial sac may also allow intrapericardial therapies with corticosteroids (e.g. intrapericardial crystalloid triamcinolone, 300 mg/m^2 body surface has been proposed for autoreactive or recurrent pericardial effusions that do not respond to other conventional therapies and in order to avoid or limit systemic side effects of corticosteroids provided orally) or antineoplastic agents.

In neoplastic pericardial effusion, most frequently due to bronchus carcinoma or breast cancer, intrapericardial cisplatin or thiotepa therapy has been proposed in combination with systemic antineoplastic treatment, which should be tailored in collaboration with the oncologist.

In rare cases of recurrent effusion, balloon pericardiotomy is an option that allows a (transient) pericardial(-pleural-)abdominal window for drainage. This approach should be avoided in neoplastic or purulent effusions to avoid the spread of the disease from the pericardium, but it is a way to prevent cardiac tamponade and improve the quality of life in oncological settings with a very poor short-term outcome [9].

An emerging application of pericardial access is electrophysiology. Pericardial access has been used for the mapping and ablation of the epicardial substrates of ventricular tachyarrhythmias with improved success rate and avoidance of a surgical procedure [11].

Key Points

- The improvements of non-invasive diagnostic tests have limited the indications for cardiac catheterization to suspected constrictive pericarditis when non-invasive imaging is inconclusive or for the assessment of cardiac tamponade during percutaneous cardiovascular interventions.
- Pericardiocentesis is indicated for cardiac tamponade and moderate to large pericardial effusions when a bacterial or neoplastic aetiology is suspected or symptomatic and non-responsive to medical therapy.
- Echocardiography and fluoroscopy allow the guidance and monitoring of pericardiocentesis.
- Additional interventional techniques include pericardioscopy, pericardial biopsy and intrapericardial therapy (steroids for recurrent pericarditis and antineoplastic agents for neoplastic pericardial effusions).

References

1. Doshi S, Ramakrishnan S, Gupta SK. Invasive hemodynamics of constrictive pericarditis. Indian Heart J. 2015;67:175–82.
2. Syed FF, Schaff HV, Oh JK. Constrictive pericarditis–a curable diastolic heart failure. Nat Rev Cardiol. 2014;11:530–44.
3. Nishimura RA, Carabello BA. Hemodynamics in the cardiac catheterization laboratory of the 21st century. Circulation. 2012;125:2138–50.
4. Sorajja P. Invasive hemodynamics of constrictive pericarditis, restrictive cardiomyopathy, and cardiac tamponade. Cardiol Clin. 2011;29:191–9.
5. Talreja DR, Nishimura RA, Oh JK, Holmes DR. Constrictive pericarditis in the modern era: novel criteria for diagnosis in the cardiac catheterization laboratory. J Am Coll Cardiol. 2008;51:315–9.
6. Loukas M, Walters A, Boon JM, Welch TP, Meiring JH, Abrahams PH. Pericardiocentesis: a clinical anatomy review. Clin Anat. 2012;25:872–81.
7. Nguyen CT, Lee E, Luo H, Siegel RJ. Echocardiographic guidance for diagnostic and therapeutic percutaneous procedures. Cardiovasc Diagn Ther. 2011;1:11–36.
8. Imazio M. Pericardial decompression syndrome: a rare but potentially fatal complication of pericardial drainage to be recognized and prevented. Eur Heart J Acute Cardiovasc Care. 2015;4:121–3.
9. Maisch B, Rupp H, Ristic A, Pankuweit S. Pericardioscopy and epi- and pericardial biopsy – a new window to the heart improving etiological diagnoses and permitting targeted intrapericardial therapy. Heart Fail Rev. 2013;18:317–28.
10. Authors/Task Force Members, Adler Y, Charron P, Imazio M, Badano L, Barón-Esquivias G, Bogaert J, Brucato A, Gueret P, Klingel K, Lionis C, Maisch B, Mayosi B, Pavie A, Ristić AD, Sabaté Tenas M, Seferovic P, Swedberg K, Tomkowski W. 2015 ESC Guidelines for the diagnosis and management of pericardial diseases: The Task Force for the Diagnosis and Management of Pericardial Diseases of the European Society of Cardiology (ESC) Endorsed by: The European Association for Cardio-Thoracic Surgery (EACTS). Eur Heart J. 2015;36:2921–64.
11. Yamada T. Transthoracic epicardial catheter ablation: indications, techniques, and complications. Circ J. 2013;77:1672–80.

Principles of Medical Therapy of Pericardial Diseases

6

6.1 Overview

The therapy of pericardial and myopericardial syndromes should be targeted as much as possible at the underlying aetiology. Nevertheless, in clinical practice, many cases remain "idiopathic", that is without a well-established aetiological diagnosis with a conventional diagnostic approach. Nothing is really "idiopathic", but in the real world, considering a cost-effective diagnostic approach, as well as the potential risks of additional invasive investigations, it may be rationale and appropriate to provide empiric medical therapies to treat the most probable diagnosis. In developed countries with a low prevalence of tuberculosis, the most common presumed aetiology is viral or immune mediated.

The conventional diagnostic approach is essentially aimed at excluding significant causes, such as bacterial infections or cancer, that may have targeted and well-established therapies. On this basis, in this chapter, it will be reviewed the mechanism of action, indications, contraindications and usual doses of main medical drugs that are used in the common clinical management of pericardial syndromes. Specific therapies will be reviewed separately for each aetiology.

6.2 Aspirin and Non-steroidal Anti-inflammatory Drugs (NSAID)

Aspirin and NSAIDs are the mainstay of the treatment of pericardial and myopericardial inflammatory syndromes (pericarditis and pericardial effusions with evidence of systemic inflammation) [1, 2].

Mechanism of Action

The primary effect of NSAIDs is the inhibition of cyclooxygenase (COX) (prostaglandin synthase), thereby impairing the ultimate transformation of

© Springer International Publishing Switzerland 2016
M. Imazio, *Myopericardial Diseases: Diagnosis and Management*,
DOI 10.1007/978-3-319-27156-9_6

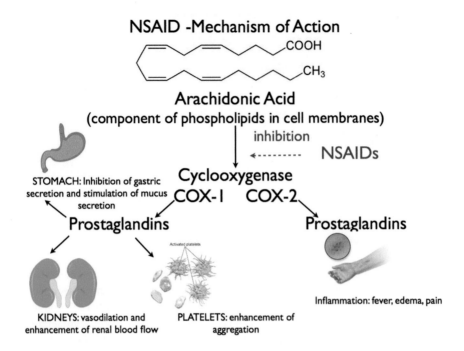

Fig. 6.1 Mechanism of action of NSAIDs. The main action is the inhibition of COX. Such effect explains the effect on inflammation and main side effects on gastrointestinal tract and kidney function

arachidonic acid to prostaglandins, prostacyclin and thromboxanes. There are two main described isoforms of COX: COX-1 and COX-2. COX-1 is expressed in most tissues and regulates normal cellular processes (such as gastric cytoprotection, vascular homeostasis, platelet aggregation and kidney function), and it is stimulated by hormones or growth factors. COX-2 is mainly expressed during inflammatory states (Fig. 6.1).

Indications

Any inflammatory pericardial syndrome.

Main Contraindications, Warnings, Precautions and Interactions

Allergy, to be used with caution in patients with platelet and bleeding disorders, dehydration and heavy ethanol use (>3 drinks/day) may increase bleeding risks and may enhance gastric mucosal damage, erosive gastritis or peptic ulcer disease and severe hepatic failure. To be used with caution in patients with mild-to-moderate renal impairment and to be avoided in severe impairment.

NSAIDs can interact with numerous drugs, including anticoagulants, antiplatelet agents, antihypertensive drugs, calcineurin inhibitors (cyclosporine and tacrolimus), digoxin, diuretics, glucocorticoids, lithium, selective serotonin reuptake inhibitors (SSRIs), methotrexate and other medications. The interaction of NSAIDs with methotrexate generally requires avoidance of NSAID use in patients receiving antineoplastic doses, while both may be used concurrently with standard doses in patients receiving low-dose methotrexate (e.g. in rheumatologic disorders).

Adverse Events

Aspirin and NSAID may affect haemostasis, thus causing bleeding. Haemorrhage may occur at virtually any site. Risk is dependent on multiple variables including dosage, concurrent use of multiple agents, which alter haemostasis, and patient susceptibility. Many adverse effects are dose related and are rare at low dosages. Other serious reactions are idiosyncratic, related to allergy or individual sensitivity. Main adverse events include agitation, confusion, dizziness, fatigue, headache, insomnia, Reye's syndrome (children), skin rash, urticaria, gastrointestinal ulcer (5–30 %), duodenal ulcer, dyspepsia, epigastric distress, gastritis, gastrointestinal erosion, heartburn, nausea, stomach pain, vomiting, anaemia, blood coagulation disorder, haemorrhage, iron deficiency anaemia, prolonged prothrombin time, thrombocytopenia, hepatitis (reversible), hepatotoxicity, increased serum transaminases, hypersensitivity (anaphylaxis, angiooedema), acetabular bone destruction, rhabdomyolysis, weakness, hearing loss, tinnitus, increased blood urea nitrogen, increased serum creatinine, interstitial nephritis, renal failure (including cases caused by rhabdomyolysis), renal insufficiency, renal papillary necrosis, asthma, bronchospasm, dyspnoea, hyperventilation, laryngeal oedema, noncardiogenic pulmonary oedema, respiratory alkalosis and tachypnea.

Special Populations

Aspirin is contraindicated in children due to the possible risk of Reye's syndrome and hepatotoxicity. Weight-adjusted doses are recommended for other NSAIDs (Table 6.1).

Aspirin can be used at lower doses during pregnancy (e.g. 500–750 mg every 8 h) before the 20 weeks and should be avoided if >20 weeks [3–7].

In the elderly, it is recommended the use of the lowest recommended doses and frequency. All patients taking aspirin and NSAIDs should receive gastroprotection with a proton pump inhibitor [4].

Common Prescribed Drugs and Dosing

In literature, the most common reported drugs include aspirin, ibuprofen and indomethacin (Fig. 6.2) [1, 2, 4].

Table 6.1 Dosing of aspirin and NSAID in children

Drug	Dosing
Aspirin	Contraindicated because of the risk of Reye's syndrome and hepatotoxicity
Ibuprofen	30–50 mg/kg/24 h divided in doses every 8 h (not to exceed the maximal dose of 2.4 g/day)
Indomethacin	To be considered for children >2 years. 1 to 2 mg/kg/day in 2–4 divided doses (not to exceed the maximal dose of 150–200 mg/day)

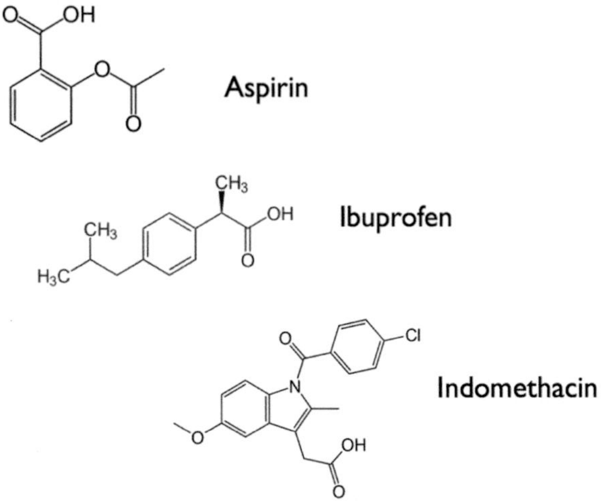

Fig. 6.2 Aspirin and commonly prescribed NSAID in pericardial syndromes

The selection of the drug should be individualized, taking into account the local availability and physician expertise, the previous history of the patient (favouring the choice of the drug proven to be most efficacious to control symptoms), concomitant therapies and disease (e.g. aspirin is the favourite choice in patients already on aspirin or with ischaemic heart disease, while corticosteroids may have less interference with patients on traditional oral anticoagulant therapy) [4].

A specific issue for clinical practice is how to use anti-inflammatory therapies in patients with ischaemic heart diseases. Aspirin should be the preferred choice in these patients: dose of aspirin up to 1500 mg/day has been demonstrated to be efficacious as antiplatelet therapy, while it is not demonstrated that higher doses (usually considered for anti-inflammatory effect) really attenuate or compromise its antiplatelet activity. Indomethacin and other NSAIDs should be avoided in patients with coronary heart disease. Most of them have a small risk of additional ischaemic events. For instance, ibuprofen and indomethacin significantly increase cardiovascular risk (RR 1–3), while naproxen (500 mg twice daily) probably is safer [8].

Additional issues to be considered are how to cope with aspirin, NSAIDs and traditional oral anticoagulant therapies. Essentially based on experts' opinion, it is advisable to use low-dose corticosteroids (e.g. prednisone 0.2–0.5 mg/kg/day) and avoid aspirin and other NSAIDs. There are no data specifically for pericardial syndromes on the use of anti-inflammatory therapies and new oral anticoagulants (e.g. dabigatran, rivaroxaban, apixaban). These statements reflect the experts' consensus provided by the 2015 European Society of Cardiology guidelines on pericardial diseases [8].

Common dosing for inflammatory pericardial syndromes is reported in Table 6.2. In order to achieve a better control of symptoms during 24 h, it is better to provide the drug every 8 h as three daily doses after meal ingestion [2, 4, 8, 9].

6.3   Colchicine

Colchicine is an ancient anti-rheumatic drug of plant origin that has been used for centuries for the treatment and prevention of gouty attacks. The term *colchicum* derives from "Colchis", an ancient region and country on the Black Sea and indicates its origin. The plant source of colchicine, the autumn crocus (*Colchicum autumnale*), was described for treatment of rheumatism and swelling in the Ebers Papyrus (ca. 1500 B.C.), an Egyptian medical papyrus (Fig. 6.3). *Colchicum* extract

Table 6.2 Common dosing of aspirin and usual NSAIDs in pericardial inflammatory syndromes	Drug	Usual dosing as initial attack dose
	Aspirin	750–1000 mg every 8 h
	Ibuprofen	600 mg every 8 h
	Indomethacin	25–50 mg every 8 h

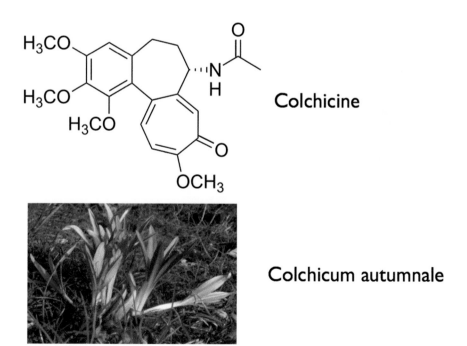

Fig. 6.3 Colchicine and its plant origin

was first described as a treatment for gout in *De Materia Medica* by Pedanius Dioscorides, in the first-century AD [10].

Mechanism of Action

The main known mechanism of action is the capability of colchicine to concentrate in white blood cells (especially granulocytes) and block tubulin polymerization thus interfering with several cellular functions (e.g. phagocytosis, degranulation, chemotaxis) that are relevant to explain its anti-inflammatory properties (Fig. 6.4).

Following the successful use of the drug to treat and prevent poliserositis attacks (including pericarditis) in patients with familial Mediterranean fever (FMF), the first idea to use colchicine for pericarditis is due to Bayes-de-Luna et al. who proposed the use of colchicine to treat and prevent recurrent pericarditis in patients without FMF in 1987. Following the successful use in single cases, prospective studies, specific trials have been planned and performed in the last 10 years, definitely showing its safety and efficacy at the proposed low doses to treat and prevent pericarditis [10].

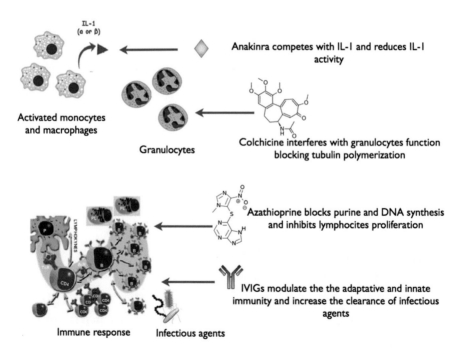

Fig. 6.4 Main mechanisms of action of colchicine and old and new emerging options for recurrent cases (azathioprine, human intravenous immunoglobulin and anakinra)

Indications

Any inflammatory pericardial syndrome to treat the acute episode. Colchicine may hasten the response to aspirin, NSAID and corticosteroids when added on top of these therapies and especially prevent recurrences.

Main Contraindications, Warnings, Precautions and Interactions

Hypersensitivity to colchicine. Colchicine should be avoided in patients with severe renal and liver impairment, pregnancy, lactation, as well as in patients with concomitant use of a strong P-glycoprotein (P-gp) or strong CYP3A4 inhibitor in presence of renal or hepatic impairment. The main drug interactions of colchicine are reported in Table 6.3.

Adverse Events

The same drug effect on the mitotic spindle may affect cells with a fast replication as those of in the gastrointestinal tract, leading to the main known side effect represented by gastrointestinal intolerance (reported in 7–10 % of cases), especially as diarrhoea but may be manifested as anorexia, nausea, vomiting, abdominal cramps and pain. Additional side effects are rare at the usual doses recommended for pericarditis (Table 6.4), fatigue (<4 %) and headache (<2 %), and in less than 1 % of cases, alopecia, bone marrow depression, dermatitis, disseminated intravascular coagulation, hepatotoxicity, hypersensitivity reaction, increased creatine phosphokinase, lactose intolerance, myalgia, myasthenia, oligospermia, purpura, rhabdomyolysis and toxic neuromuscular disease [10].

In clinical trials, the use of colchicine on top of standard anti-inflammatory therapies increases the risks of side effects (mainly diarrhoea: OR 1.45, 95 % CI 1.04–2.03) and drug discontinuation (OR 1.40, 95 % CI 1.00–1.94) [11, 12].

Special Populations

Doses reduction by 50 % is warranted in children and elderly (>65 years). In the absence of a major clinical indication (e.g. familial Mediterranean fever attacks prevention), colchicine is contraindicated during pregnancy and lactation [8, 10].

Common Dosing

Results of meta-analyses from randomized trials confirm its efficacy for the secondary prevention of pericarditis after a first attack (OR 0.31 95 % CI 0.19–0.52) and

Table 6.3 Major contraindications and interactions of colchicine

Feature	Data
Major contraindications	Concomitant use of a P-glycoprotein (P-gp) or strong CYP3A4 inhibitor in presence of renal or hepatic impairment
	Severe renal impairment
	Severe liver disease
	Pregnancy
Major interactions	*HMG-CoA reductase inhibitors*: Colchicine may enhance the myopathic (rhabdomyolysis) effect of *HMG-CoA reductase Inhibitors*. Colchicine may increase the serum concentration of *HMG-CoA reductase inhibitors*
	Strong CYP3A4 inhibitor (e.g. *clarithromycin, itraconazole, ketoconazole, cyclosporine*): May increase the serum concentration of colchicine. Management: Colchicine is contraindicated in patients with impaired renal or hepatic function who are also receiving a strong CYP3A4 inhibitor. In those with normal renal and hepatic function, reduce colchicine dose, generally by 50 %. Careful monitoring, consider co-morbidities
	P-gp inhibitor (e.g. *cyclosporine, ranolazine*): May increase the serum concentration of colchicine. Colchicine distribution into certain tissues (e.g., brain) may also be increased. Management: Colchicine is contraindicated in patients with impaired renal or hepatic function who are also receiving a p-glycoprotein inhibitor. In those with normal renal and hepatic function, reduce colchicine dose by 50 %. Careful monitoring, consider co-morbidities
Dose adjustment:	
Children <5 years	Reduce daily dose by 50 %
Elderly >65–70 years	Reduce daily dose by 50 %
Renal failure:	CrCl 30–60 mL/min: Monitor closely for adverse effects; dose reduction by 50 %
–	CrCl 15–30 mL/min: Initial dose: 0.5 mg every 2 days; monitor for adverse effects
	Dialysis or CrCl <15 mL/min: do not use

after multiple recurrences (OR 0.31 95 % CI 0.19–0.52) (LOE A) [11]. On this basis colchicine has a Class I indication, LOE A according to 2015 ESC guidelines [8].

Colchicine should be added on top of standard anti-inflammatory therapy (aspirin/NSAID or corticosteroid) in order to fasten the response to therapy and reduce the risk of subsequent recurrences generally by 50 %. The drug is provided at weight-adjusted doses (e.g. 0.5 mg twice daily or once daily in those <70 kg and impaired renal function) without a loading dose to improve its tolerability (Table 6.4) [8, 9].

Monitoring of disease activity is based on weekly assessment of C-reactive protein. Safety monitoring of treatment is performed with assessment of symptoms and signs related to toxicity and chemistry assessment (essentially transaminases,

Table 6.4 Dosing and monitoring of colchicine for pericardial inflammatory syndromes

Drug	Attack dose	Treatment length
Colchicine	0.5 mg twice daily (>70 kg), or 0.5 mg if weight <70 kg	3 months (acute) 6–12 months (recurrent)

creatine kinase, blood count, creatinine) at least at 1 month and then according to clinical evolution, potential interfering drugs.

6.4 Corticosteroids

Corticosteroids are generally successful to achieve a fast control of symptoms and reduction of pericardial effusion but are associated with a prolonged course and more recurrences especially if used at high doses (e.g. prednisone 1.0 mg/kg/day or equivalent) (LOE B) [5].

Mechanism of Action

Corticosteroids are steroidal hormones that enter cells and combine with steroid receptors in cytoplasm and then enter the nucleus and control the synthesis of proteins, including enzymes that regulate vital cells activity, several metabolic functions and inflammation. Moreover they inhibit the enzyme phospholipase A2 thus blocking the supply of arachidonic acid for the synthesis of prostaglandins, thromboxane A2 and leukotrienes (Fig. 6.5). As a result of the action of corticosteroids, the inflammatory response is depressed, as well as allergic responses, lymphoid tissue and antibodies production.

Indications

Corticosteroids should be considered only as second-line drugs or for specific indications (e.g. contraindications or severe intolerance to NSAIDs and aspirin, systemic inflammatory diseases on steroids or requiring such therapy, pregnancy, uremic pericarditis and failure of first-line treatments) [8] (Figs. 6.6 and 6.7).

Adverse Events

In a specific retrospective study on recurrent pericarditis, high doses of prednisone (1.0 mg/kg/day) were associated with severe side effects, recurrences and hospitalizations (hazard ratio, 3.61; 95 % confidence interval, 1.96–6.63; $P<0.001$) compared with lower dose (prednisone 0.2–0.5 mg/kg/day) and also after adjustment for potential confounders (age, female gender, non-idiopathic origin). Especially high

Mechanisms of Action of Corticosteroids

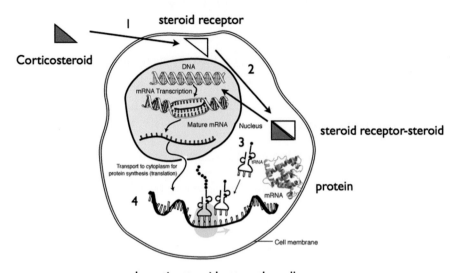

1: corticosteroid enters the cell
2: binding to intracytoplasmatic receptor
3. induction of gene expression and protein synthesis
4. protein synthesis

Fig. 6.5 Mechanism of action of corticosteroids inducing protein synthesis. *1* Corticosteroid enters the cell. *2* Binding to intracytoplasmic receptor. *3* Induction of gene expression and protein synthesis. *4* Protein synthesis

doses are associated with severe side effects (up to 25 % of cases frequently leading to drug withdrawal) [5]. The reported side effects include increased appetite, acne, mood changes and mental health problems (depression, anxiety, insomnia), muscle weakness, a combination of fatty deposits in the face, stretch marks across the body (the so-called Cushing's syndrome), osteoporosis, diabetes, systemic arterial hypertension, glaucoma and cataract, increased risk of infections and impaired growth in children. All these side effects have been reported in patients with recurrent and chronic forms following prolonged therapies with corticosteroids.

Special Populations

Corticosteroids can be used in children, where the use should be limited for the possible effects on growth and additional side effects. Steroids have no contraindications in pregnancy. In the elderly, the use of steroids should be cautious because of an increased risk of side effects. Bisphosphonates are recommended to prevent bone loss in all men ≥50 years and postmenopausal women in

Prednisone and Corticosteroids

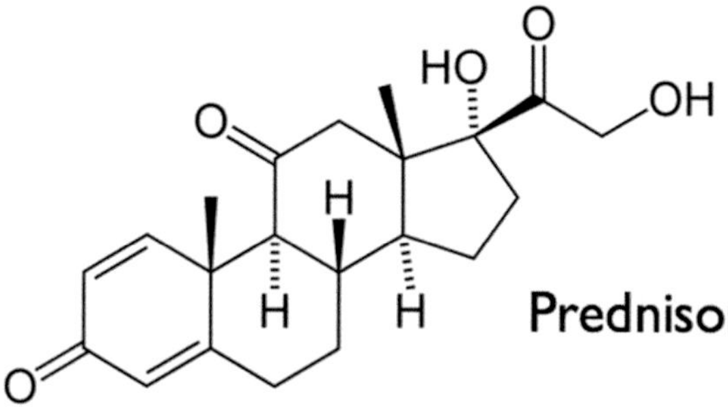

Prednisone

Steroid	Anti-inflammatory potency	Sodium retention potency	Duration (hours)	Equivalent dose (mg)
Cortisol	1	1	8-12	20
Cortisone	0.8	0.8	8-12	25
Fludrocortisone	10	12.5	8-12	na
Prednisone	4	0.8	12-36	5
Prednisolone	4	0.8	12-36	5
Methylprednisolone	5	0.5	12-36	4
Triamcinolone	5	0	12-36	4
Betamethasone	25	0	36-72	0.75
Dexamethasone	25	0	36-72	0.75

Fig. 6.6 Prednisone and other corticosteroids with equivalent dosing

whom long-term treatment with glucocorticoids is initiated at a dose ≥5.0–7.5 mg/ day of prednisone or equivalent [8].

Common Dosing

Corticosteroids should be used at low to moderate doses (e.g. prednisone 0.2–0.5 mg/kg/day or equivalent, Figs. 6.6 and 6.7) with colchicine till symptoms resolution and normalization of markers of inflammation with a slow tapering [1, 2, 5, 8].

A slow tapering (e.g. to decrease the dose of prednisone by 1.0–2.5 mg every 2–4 weeks in particular at the critical dose threshold for recurrences) is critical, and each tapering should be considered only in asymptomatic patients after normalization of CRP. A slower tapering with 1 mg instead of 2.5 mg is a useful option especially in cases with additional recurrences with 2.5 mg-tapering (Table 6.5) [5].

Five major indications to corticosteroids in pericardial diseases

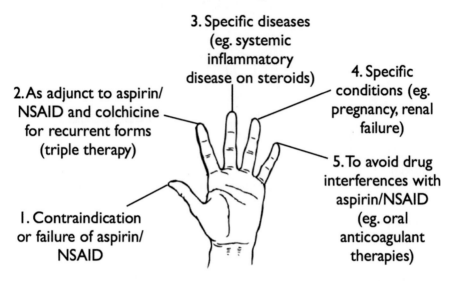

Fig. 6.7 The specific indications for corticosteroid therapy in pericardial diseases (the exceptions to the general rule to avoid them as first line therapy)

Table 6.5 Suggested tapering of prednisone in pericardial inflammatory syndromes

Prednisone dose[a]	Starting dose 0.25–0.50 mg/kg/day[a]	Tapering[b]
Prednisone daily dose	>50 mg	10 mg/day every 1–2 weeks
	50–25 mg	5–10 mg/day every 1–2 weeks
	25–15 mg	2.5 mg/day every 2–4 weeks
	<15 mg	1.25–2.5 mg/day every 2–6 weeks

Calcium intake (supplement plus oral intake) 1,200–1,500 mg/day and vitamin D supplementation 800–1000 IU/day should be offered to all patients receiving glucocorticoids
[a]Avoid higher doses except for special cases and only for a few days, with rapid tapering to 25 mg/day. Prednisone 25 mg is equivalent to methylprednisolone 20 mg
[b]Every decrease in prednisone dose should be done only if the patient is asymptomatic and C-reactive protein is normal, particularly for doses <25 mg/day

6.5   Azathioprine, Human Intravenous Immunoglobulin (IVIG) and Anakinra

In patients with refractory recurrent episodes, alternative treatments beyond aspirin, NSAIDs, colchicine and corticosteroids have been evaluated. Among the most promising old and new emerging treatments, the three most common and evidence-based therapies are: azathioprine, human intravenous immunoglobulin (IVIG) and

Table 6.6   Azathioprine, IVIG and anakinra dosing

Drug	Dosing
Azathioprine	Starting with 1 mg/kg day then gradually increased to 2–3 mg/kg/day for several months
IVIG	400–500 mg iv daily for 5 days
Anakinra	1–2 mg/kg/day up to 100 mg/day in adults for several months

anakinra (Table 6.6) [13]. The main mechanism of action of each drug is reported in Fig. 6.4.

Azathioprine

Azathioprine is an immunosuppressive drug belonging to the chemical class of purine analogues that is commonly used in organ transplantation recipients and autoimmune diseases. NSAIDs and corticosteroids may be combined and continued, and the drug is especially a steroid-sparing agent to reduce and withdraw corticosteroids with a slow onset of action (1–2 months) that requires a prolonged therapy of several months [13]. The largest reported experience is a single-centre, retrospective study of 46 patients with idiopathic recurrent pericarditis (mean age 40 years, range 11–71 years), where azathioprine was administered at the dose of 1.5–2.5 mg/kg die for 13.6 ± 5.1 months in the idiopathic forms. The use of azathioprine was associated with stable remission following steroid discontinuation in more than 50 % of patients [14]. Liver toxicity and myelosuppression are the most feared complications of this therapy; they are generally dose dependent and usually resolve in 7–10 days with dose reduction or discontinuation. However, the risk of myelodysplastic syndrome cannot be excluded and requires careful long-term monitoring. Overall azathioprine was well tolerated in the mentioned study: transient hepatotoxicity was observed in about 10 % of cases and leucopenia in 6–7 %; transient gastrointestinal symptoms with spontaneous resolution were reported in 4–5 % of cases.

Overall, azathioprine is a potentially useful, cheap and safe solution in patients who do not respond to conventional therapies and are not able to withdraw corticosteroids (LOE C) [8]. Azathioprine is essentially a steroid-sparing agent useful in the long run; it is less useful in the resolution of an acute attack. The recommended initial dosage is 1 mg/kg/day given once daily, gradually increased till 2–3 mg/kg/day. Concomitant therapy with allopurinol greatly increases bone marrow toxicity and must be avoided [8].

Intravenous Immunoglobulins (IVIG)

IVIGs are prepared from plasma pooled from healthy donors. Administered IVIGs can exert both anti-inflammatory and immunomodulatory effects; moreover they may be helpful for the clearance of infectious agents [13, 15]. This treatment has been studied both in children and adults with recurrent pericarditis with limited published data [16–18]. Overall, IVIG are a possible rapidly acting, safe and efficacious steroid-sparing treatment for refractory pericarditis (LOE C), useful in the management of the acute attack; recurrences may occur after IVIG discontinuation. The main limitations of this treatment are represented by the costs (rather expensive and hospitalization or day hospital facility may be required for administration) and possible safety concerns related to the need of administration of plasma derivate from "healthy donors" [16–18].

Anakinra and Biological Agents

Anakinra is a recombinant form of the naturally occurring interleukin-1 (IL-1) receptor antagonist that has been successfully used in patients with FMF after colchicine failure. It is a biologic response modifier that acts by antagonizing the biologic effects of IL-1, which is a proinflammatory cytokine [13]. It is currently approved by the Food and Drug Administration for the treatment of rheumatoid arthritis. The drug has been initially used in paediatric patients, where the long-term side effects of corticosteroids are particularly relevant, such as the deleterious effects on growth, and also in adult patients with refractory recurrent pericarditis, especially if corticosteroid-dependent [19–23]. Anakinra is a potentially useful, effective, rapidly acting steroid-sparing agent (LOE C). However, recurrences after drug discontinuation are a matter of concern, and the drug is rather expensive. RCTs are required to confirm these findings and address the most effective treatment protocol [23].

> **Key Points**
> - Aspirin and non-steroidal drugs (NSAID) are mainstay of empiric anti-inflammatory therapy for pericardial diseases.
> - Colchicine is an adjunct on top of this empiric anti-inflammatory therapy to fasten the response, improve remission rates and halve recurrences.
> - Corticosteroids are a second-level option to be considered at low to moderate doses (e.g. prednisone 0.2–0.5 mg/kg/day) in case of contraindications or failure of aspirin/NSAID and for specific indications (e.g. pregnancy, systemic inflammatory diseases with an indication to corticosteroids).
> - For refractory cases, new emerging options are represented by azathioprine, human intravenous immunoglobulins and biological agents such as anakinra.

References

1. Imazio M, Adler Y. Treatment with aspirin, NSAID, corticosteroids, and colchicine in acute and recurrent pericarditis. Heart Fail Rev. 2013;18:355–60.
2. Imazio M, et al. Medical therapy of pericardial diseases: part II: noninfectious pericarditis, pericardial effusion and constrictive pericarditis. J Cardiovasc Med (Hagerstown). 2010;11:785–94.

3. Lotrionte M, et al. International collaborative systematic review of controlled clinical trials on pharmacologic treatments for acute pericarditis and its recurrences. Am Heart J. 2010;160:662–70.
4. Imazio M, Brucato A, Trinchero R, Spodick D, Adler Y. Individualized therapy for pericarditis. Expert Rev Cardiovasc Ther. 2009;7:965–75.
5. Imazio M, Brucato A, Cumetti D, Brambilla G, Demichelis B, Ferro S, Maestroni S, Cecchi E, Belli R, Palmieri G, Trinchero R. Corticosteroids for recurrent pericarditis: high versus low doses: a nonrandomized observation. Circulation. 2008;118:667–71.
6. Ristić AD, et al. Pericardial disease in pregnancy. Herz. 2003;28:209–15.
7. Imazio M, et al. Management of pericardial diseases during pregnancy. J Cardiovasc Med (Hagerstown). 2010;11:557–62.
8. Authors/Task Force Members; Adler Y, Charron P, Imazio M, Badano L, Barón-Esquivias G, Bogaert J, Brucato A, Gueret P, Klingel K, Lionis C, Maisch B, Mayosi B, Pavie A, Ristić AD, Sabaté Tenas M, Seferovic P, Swedberg K, Tomkowski W. 2015 ESC Guidelines for the diagnosis and management of pericardial diseases: The Task Force for the Diagnosis and Management of Pericardial Diseases of the European Society of Cardiology (ESC)Endorsed by: The European Association for Cardio-Thoracic Surgery (EACTS). Eur Heart J. 2015;36:2921–64.
9. Imazio M. New clinical trials in acute and recurrent pericarditis. Curr Cardiol Rep. 2015;17:23.
10. Imazio M. Colchicine for pericarditis. Trends Cardiovasc Med. 2015;25:129–36.
11. Briasoulis A, Afonso L. Prevention of pericarditis with colchicine: an updated meta-analysis. J Cardiovasc Med (Hagerstown). 2015;16:144–7.
12. Alabed S, Cabello JB, Irving GJ, Qintar M, Burls A. Colchicine for pericarditis. Cochrane Database Syst Rev. 2014;8:CD010652.
13. Imazio M, Lazaros G, Brucato A, Gaita F. Recurrent pericarditis: new and emerging therapeutic options. Nat Rev Cardiol. 2015. doi:10.1038/nrcardio.2015.115. [Epub ahead of print].
14. Vianello F, et al. Azathioprine in isolated recurrent pericarditis: a single centre experience. Int J Cardiol. 2011;147:477–8.
15. Gelfand EW. Intravenous immune globulin in autoimmune and inflammatory diseases. N Engl J Med. 2012;367:2015–25.
16. del Fresno MR, Peralta JE, Granados MÁ, Enríquez E, Domínguez-Pinilla N, de Inocencio J. Intravenous immunoglobulin therapy for refractory recurrent pericarditis. Pediatrics. 2014;134:e1441–6.
17. Moretti M, et al. Usefulness of high-dose intravenous human immunoglobulins treatment for refractory recurrent pericarditis. Am J Cardiol. 2013;112:1493–8.
18. Imazio M, et al. Intravenous human immunoglobulins for refractory recurrent pericarditis. A systematic review of all published cases. J Cardiovasc Med (Hagerstown). 2015. [Epub ahead of print].
19. Grattagliano I, et al. Novel therapeutics for the treatment of familial Mediterranean fever: from colchicine to biologics. Clin Pharmacol Ther. 2014;95:89–97.
20. Mertens M, Singh JA. Anakinra for rheumatoid arthritis: a systematic review. J Rheumatol. 2009;36:1118–25.
21. Picco P, et al. Successful treatment of idiopathic recurrent pericarditis in children with interleukin-1beta receptor antagonist (anakinra): an unrecognized autoinflammatory disease? Arthritis Rheum. 2009;60:264–8.
22. Lazaros G, et al. Anakinra for the management of resistant idiopathic recurrent pericarditis. Initial experience in 10 adult cases. Ann Rheum Dis. 2014;73:2215–7.
23. Lazaros G, et al. Anakinra: an emerging option for refractory idiopathic recurrent pericarditis. A systematic review of published evidence. J Cardiovasc Med (Hagerstown). 2015. [Epub ahead of print].

Surgery for Pericardial Diseases

7

7.1 Introduction

Under a surgical point of view, the different pathological pericardial entities may be grouped into non-constrictive, constrictive pericardial diseases and tumours (Fig. 7.1) [1].

7.2 Non-constrictive Pericardial Diseases

Non-constrictive pericardial diseases of surgical interest include pericardial effusions.

Whenever a large pericardial effusion cannot be adequately drained percutaneously, surgical drainage is advisable (e.g. purulent effusion, loculated effusions, recurrent pericardial effusions not responding to medical therapy) and can be achieved by *mediastinal exploration* (in case of uncontrollable bleeding or in the presence of a concomitant cardiac disease that requires intracardiac repair and mediastinal exploration) or creation of a *pericardial window* [1].

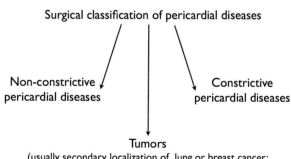

Surgical classification of pericardial diseases

Non-constrictive pericardial diseases

Constrictive pericardial diseases

Tumors
(usually secondary localization of lung or breast cancer; primary disease is rare (mainly mesothelioma)

Fig. 7.1 Surgical classification of pericardial diseases

© Springer International Publishing Switzerland 2016
M. Imazio, *Myopericardial Diseases: Diagnosis and Management*,
DOI 10.1007/978-3-319-27156-9_7

Pericardial Window

A *pericardial window* is a cardiac surgical procedure to create a communication – or "window" – from the pericardial space. Drainage can be performed directly through a *subxiphoid approach* or indirectly into the pleural space or peritoneal cavity after pericardiotomy (the most common approach is the *transpleural approach* that can be achieved by either lateral thoracotomy or video-assisted thoracoscopy). During the procedure pericardial biopsy can be performed for the study of pericardial tissue [1].

A pericardial window by subxiphoid approach is usually done through a vertical lower chest incision, then the rectus abdominis is divided through the linea alba and the xiphoid process is exposed and incised or retracted (Fig. 7.2). After the incision of the pericardium, pericardial drainage is performed, and a single 24–32 F chest tube is placed.

The procedure is generally performed with general anaesthesia, and it is especially useful in case of infections in order to prevent the spread of the infection and pleural empyema (e.g. purulent pericarditis). However, a limitation of this approach is to gain a temporary drainage of pericardial space.

In case of persistent or recurrent pericardial effusions, a better option is to consider a pericardial window by a transpleural approach either by lateral thoracotomy or video-assisted thoracoscopy. A left side approach is usually favoured because more pericardium is present on the left side in levocardia. The procedure is completed through the insertion of 1 or 2 chest tubes in the pleural space. The thoracoscopic approach is less invasive but requires single lung ventilation.

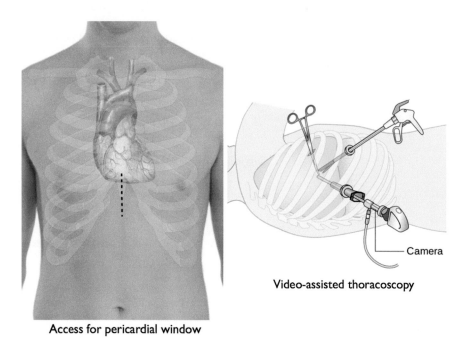

Camera

Video-assisted thoracoscopy

Access for pericardial window

Fig. 7.2 Access for pericardial window and video-assisted thoracoscopy (Modified from Cancer Research UK/Wikimedia Commons)

The purpose of the window is to allow a pericardial effusion (usually malignant) to drain from the space surrounding the heart into the chest cavity – in order to prevent large pericardial effusion and cardiac tamponade.

The creation of pericardial windows allows avoidance of a more complex operation, such as pericardiectomy, when there is a high surgical risk or the life expectancy of the patients is reduced (e.g. neoplastic pericardial disease) and the intervention is palliative. The results of a pericardial window are less definitive and recurrence may occur.

For recurrent pericardial effusion not responsive to medical therapy, a last option that can be offered is *complete pericardiectomy*, usually with a good outcome and very limited perioperative complications [1].

7.3   Constrictive Pericardial Diseases

The presence of permanent constriction is a clear indication for pericardiectomy.

Pericardiectomy may be *complete or radical* with the complete removal of the whole pericardium. A total removal is not possible since small strips of the pericardium need to be preserved with phrenic nerves, but in this case, the surgeon starts removing the anterior pericardium (from phrenic nerve to phrenic nerve), followed by the diaphragmatic pericardium (Fig. 7.3), and then the pericardium posterior to the left phrenic nerve (Fig. 7.4) [1].

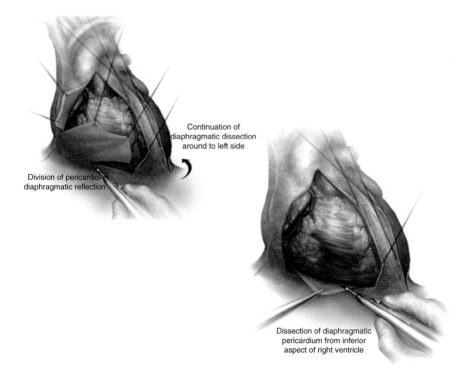

Fig. 7.3 First steps in total pericardiectomy with removal of the anterior pericardium and then the diaphragmatic pericardium (Reproduced with permission from Cho and Schaff [1])

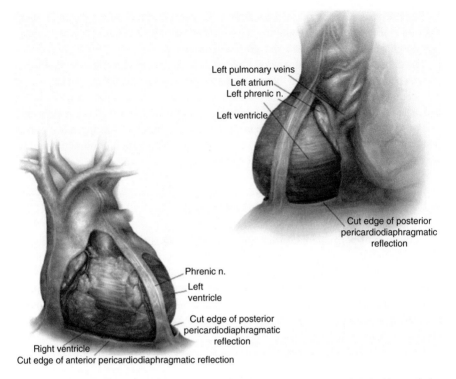

Left pulmonary veins
Left atrium
Left phrenic n.

Left ventricle

Cut edge of posterior
pericardiodiaphragmatic
reflection

Phrenic n.

Left
ventricle

Cut edge of posterior
pericardiodiaphragmatic
reflection

Right ventricle
Cut edge of anterior pericardiodiaphragmatic reflection

Fig. 7.4 Removal of the pericardium posterior to the left phrenic nerve (Reproduced with permission from Cho and Schaff [1])

Partial pericardiectomy, also named *anterior pericardiectomy*, is the removal of the anterior pericardium from the right phrenic nerve to the left phrenic nerve. This surgical operation is easier, avoiding the exposition of the inferior and left lateral surfaces of the ventricles, and moreover is able to improve the haemodynamic of most patients. However, incomplete results and recurrences of constriction are possible and may require an additional surgical operation. In most institutions, total or radical pericardiectomy is the surgical operation of choice for patients with constrictive pericarditis. Cardiopulmonary bypass is not necessary for all patients but may help since decompression of the heart with extracorporeal circulation may help to dissect and manipulate the ventricles as well as to repair possible injuries of the myocardium. In these patients, cardiopulmonary bypass and systemic heparinization increase the bleeding risk.

An important issue is to check for adequate removal of any residual epicardial constriction that can be easily verified by observing the expansion of the ventricles after complete removal of the constrictive pericardium.

Results of this surgery are good, and in current era the in-hospital mortality ranges from 5 to 10 %. Age, advanced disease and especially the aetiology of constriction are main mortality predictors. Radiation constrictive pericarditis has the worse outcomes since fibrosis involves the myocardium, valves, coronary arteries as well as lungs and chest. In patients with more advanced disease, tricuspid regurgitation may be present and may worsen after removal of the pericardium, thus requiring valve repair. Intraoperative transoesophageal echocardiography is essential to monitor tricuspid valve function during the operation. Tricuspid valve repair is advisable also in those with moderate to severe tricuspid regurgitation before pericardiectomy [1].

Pericardiectomy is the definite surgical operation for patients with permanent constrictive pericarditis. However, the identification of transient form related to pericardial inflammation should suggest caution in any acute, new-onset form of constrictive pericarditis. In such patients, potentially reversible forms of constriction may occur and an empiric trial of anti-inflammatory therapy is warranted waiting at least 3 months before resorting to pericardiectomy in those with persistent constriction. The identification of the reversible cases can be helped by the identification of inflammatory signs on imaging (e.g. pericardial oedema and late gadolinium enhancement on cardiac magnetic resonance) and/or in blood (e.g. elevation of C-reactive protein) [2–4].

Key Points
- Under a surgical point of view, pericardial diseases can be divided into constrictive and non-constrictive diseases.
- The definite therapy for permanent chronic constriction is radical pericardiectomy.
- New-onset forms of constrictive pericarditis may be provoked by pericardial inflammation and may be transient and reversible with anti-inflammatory therapy.
- Empiric anti-inflammatory therapy should be considered in these cases with possible transient constriction if there is evidence of elevation of markers of systemic inflammation or pericardial inflammation on imaging (CT or CMR).
- Total pericardiectomy may be considered for refractory recurrent pericarditis after failure of medical therapy.

References

1. Cho YH, Schaff HV. Surgery for pericardial disease. Heart Fail Rev. 2013;18(3):375–87.
2. Feng D, Glockner J, Kim K, Martinez M, Syed IS, Araoz P, Breen J, Espinosa RE, Sundt T, Schaff HV, Oh JK. Cardiac magnetic resonance imaging pericardial late gadolinium enhancement and elevated inflammatory markers can predict the reversibility of constrictive pericarditis after antiinflammatory medical therapy: a pilot study. Circulation. 2011;124:1830–7.
3. Seferović PM, Ristić AD, Maksimović R, Simeunović DS, Milinković I, Seferović Mitrović JP, Kanjuh V, Pankuweit S, Maisch B. Pericardial syndromes: an update after the ESC guidelines 2004. Heart Fail Rev. 2013;18:255–66.
4. Azam S, Hoit BD. Treatment of pericardial disease. Cardiovasc Ther. 2011;29:308–14.

Part II

Myopericardial Syndromes

Pericardial Syndromes

8

Different aetiological agents either infectious or non-infectious (see chapter on the aetiology of pericardial diseases) interact with the pericardium in a rather non-specific way causing inflammation of the pericardium (pericarditis) with possible increased production of pericardial fluid or in some cases reduced reabsorption (pericardial effusion) [1–3]. The pericardium is rather rigid, and sudden changes of its volume may occur only with sudden increase of intrapericardial pressure generating a compressing effect on cardiac chambers and impairing diastolic filling during the entire diastole, thus causing a reduced cardiac output (cardiac tamponade) [3]. On the contrary, slowly accumulating pericardial fluid may occur without the development of cardiac tamponade in other cases (isolate chronic large pericardial effusion) [3]. The final stage of any pathological process affecting the pericardium is represented by fibrosis with possible thickening and calcification leading to a loss of pericardial elasticity and a constrictive effect of the pericardium on cardiac chambers, thus impairing diastolic filling in mid-late diastole (constrictive pericarditis).

In clinical practice, all these manifestation of pericardial disease can be grouped in specific presentations including signs and symptoms and having peculiar diagnostic, therapeutic and prognostic features. Such distinct clinical presentations are usually named "pericardial syndromes" [4–6]. The main pericardial syndromes include:

1. Acute and recurrent pericarditis
2. Pericardial effusion
3. Cardiac tamponade
4. Constrictive pericarditis
5. Pericardial masses and cysts
6. Congenital abnormalities of the pericardium

The main syndromes are linked together, and one may progress into the other, being the last chronic step, generally constrictive pericarditis, as final common way for different initial causes (e.g. infections, trauma, cardiac surgery, radiation) (Fig. 8.1) [5–7].

© Springer International Publishing Switzerland 2016
M. Imazio, *Myopericardial Diseases: Diagnosis and Management*,
DOI 10.1007/978-3-319-27156-9_8

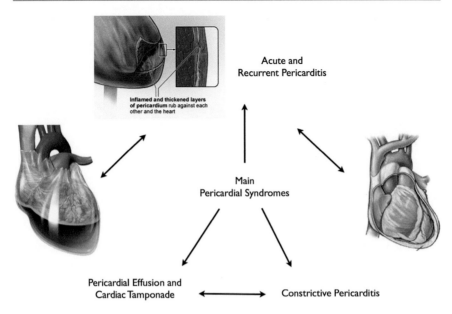

Fig. 8.1 Main pericardial syndromes (see text for explanation)

In the next chapters, each syndrome will be reviewed in order to provide the best evidence-based management in clinical practice.

References

1. LeWinter MM. Clinical practice. Acute pericarditis. N Engl J Med. 2014;371:2410–6.
2. Lilly LS. Treatment of acute and recurrent idiopathic pericarditis. Circulation. 2013;127: 1723–6.
3. Imazio M, Adler Y. Management of pericardial effusion. Eur Heart J. 2013;34:1186–97.
4. Seferović PM, Ristić AD, Maksimović R, Simeunović DS, Milinković I, Seferović Mitrović JP, Kanjuh V, Pankuweit S, Maisch B. Pericardial syndromes: an update after the ESC guidelines 2004. Heart Fail Rev. 2013;18:255–66.
5. Peebles CR, Shambrook JS, Harden SP. Pericardial disease – anatomy and function. Br J Radiol. 2011;84 Spec No 3:S324–37.
6. Imazio M. Contemporary management of pericardial diseases. Curr Opin Cardiol. 2012;27:308–17.
7. Dudzinski DM, Mak GS, Hung JW. Pericardial diseases. Curr Probl Cardiol. 2012;37:75–118.

Acute Pericarditis: Management Overview

9

9.1 Definition

Acute pericarditis is the most common pericardial syndrome that is encountered in clinical practice. It is an inflammatory pericardial syndrome with or without pericardial effusion [1, 2].

9.2 Presentation

The usual presentation is acute, with *retrosternal "chest pain" with pleuritic features* (>85 % of cases; it is increased by inspiration), and it has positional features: worsening when the patient is supine and improves when sitting and leaning forward. It may radiate to the shoulders, arms and jaw and may simulate "ischaemic chest pain". It is a typical "referred pain" since pericardial afferent fibres show convergence with somatic areas on the chest and arms as for angina pain (Fig. 9.1) [1, 2].

The physical examination may be normal; patients may have a low-degree fever in uncomplicated cases and additional signs and symptoms related to a concomitant febrile syndrome (e.g. gastroenteritis, flu-like syndrome that may also precede pericarditis 1–2 weeks before) or an underlying disease with pericardial involvement (e.g. systemic inflammatory disease, cancer). The most specific physical sign can be the presence of a *pericardial rub* that is identifiable in no more than 1 of 3 cases. It is a superficial scratchy or squeaking sound best heard with the diaphragm of the stethoscope over the left sternal border and better with the patient sitting up and leaning forward. It is typically compared with the sound produced by walking on fresh snow and it can be evanescent [2–4].

On ECG, the classical reported feature of acute pericarditis is *widespread ST-segment elevation* (Fig. 9.2), although either this sign or the earlier *PR depression* (as an atrial current of injury that is the earliest ECG sign) is the expression of concomitant subepicardial involvement and not "pure pericarditis", since the pericardium is electrically silent [3, 5].

© Springer International Publishing Switzerland 2016
M. Imazio, *Myopericardial Diseases: Diagnosis and Management*,
DOI 10.1007/978-3-319-27156-9_9

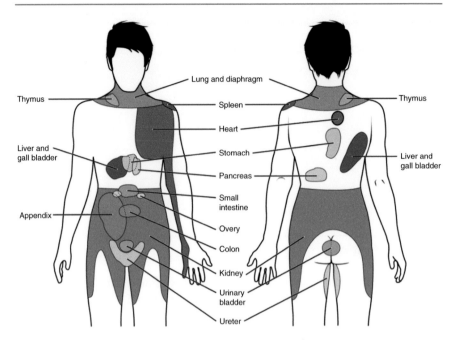

Fig. 9.1 Pericardial pain as a referred pain with features common with anginal pain. The convergence of afferent sensitive pathways from both visceral organs (heart and pericardium) and cutaneous area is responsible for the difficulty of the central nervous system to discern the two types of pain; thus visceral pain may be referred to an area of the thorax (restrosternal) and arms, especially the left arm (Reproduced from *Autonomic Reflexes and Homeostasis* http://cnx.org/content/m46579/1.2/, by OpenStax College)

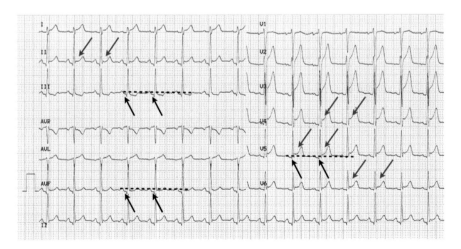

Fig. 9.2 Classical ECG with "widespread ST-segment elevation" (see red arrows) and PR depression (see black arrows) in a young patient with acute pericarditis

Fig. 9.3 Chest x-ray in a
young patient with acute
pericarditis with normal
findings

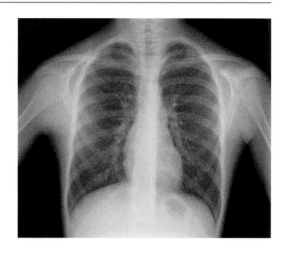

A so-called "typical" ECG can be found in no more than 60 % of cases and ST/T changes are more common in younger male patients, especially with associated myocarditis. The ECG evolves according to classical 4 stages reported by Spodick et al. in no more than 60 %. Presentation times as well as therapies may affect the ECG presentation. Early presentation may show ST-segment elevation, on the contrary a normal ECG or with negative T waves (reflecting an ECG in evolution) can be seen in late presentations or chronic forms. In patients with a fast response to medical therapy, the ECG may be absolutely normal as well as in mild forms; thus, a normal ECG does not exclude pericarditis [2, 5]. The risk of cardiac arrhythmias is very low in simple acute pericarditis, that is, in the absence of myocarditis or structural heart diseases [3, 6].

Chest x-ray may be completely normal (Fig. 9.3) in the absence of concomitant pleuropulmonary disease or large pericardial effusion (>300 ml).

An echocardiogram is mandatory in a patient with a suspicion of acute pericarditis to assess the presence, size and haemodynamic importance of pericardial effusion. About 60 % of patients with acute pericarditis will show a pericardial effusion, generally mild [4]. Alternatively, it is common to find non-specific increase of pericardial brightness, probably related to fibrinous exudation in pericardial layers (Fig. 9.4). On this basis, also the absence of a pericardial effusion does not exclude pericarditis.

All the symptoms and signs are due to inflamed pericardial layers with increased attrition (pericardial pain, rubs), possible increased production of pericardial effusion (pericardial effusion) and subepicardial inflammatory involvement (ECG changes, concomitant myocarditis) (See also Fig. 3.5 in Chap. 3).

Chemistry may show elevation of markers of inflammation in most cases (e.g. elevation of C-reactive protein and white blood cells count) but not all because of a possible early presentation or effect of empiric anti-inflammatory therapies; thus, normal markers of inflammations do not exclude pericarditis [7].

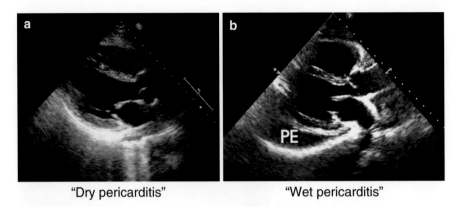

"Dry pericarditis"   "Wet pericarditis"

Fig. 9.4 Panel (**a**) A patient with "dry" acute pericarditis with increased brightness of pericardial layers, a non-specific echocardiographic sign. Panel (**b**) A patient with acute pericarditis and a moderate (10–20 mm of telediastolic echo-free space) pericardial effusion

9.3   Aetiology and Diagnosis

The aetiology of acute pericarditis largely depends on the prevalence of tuberculosis. In developed areas with a low prevalence of tuberculosis (e.g. Western Europe and North America), most cases are presumed to be viral and usually preceded or concomitant with a flu-like syndrome or gastroenteritis [1, 7, 8]. The most common viral agents, which may be also responsible for myocarditis, include *Enteroviruses* (especially Coxsackieviruses), herpes viruses (especially Epstein-Barr virus (EBV) and reactivation of cytomegalovirus (CMV)), parvovirus and only in a minority of cases influenza viruses, HCV and HBV. In children either *Enteroviruses* or *Adenoviruses* or herpes viruses are implicated [1, 2]. Nevertheless, in clinical practice most cases remain "idiopathic" with a conventional diagnostic approach and account for about 85 % of cases. In developing countries, tuberculosis is the most common cause of pericarditis and pericardial diseases, and it is often associated with HIV infection, especially in specific geographic areas, such as sub-Saharan Africa (Table 9.1) [9].

The clinical diagnosis can be made *with two of the following criteria* (Table 9.2) [2, 10, 11]:

1. Chest pain
2. Pericardial friction rub
3. Electrocardiographic (ECG) changes with new widespread ST elevation or PR depression in the acute phase
4. Pericardial effusion (new or worsening)

In case of atypical or doubtful presentation, elevation of markers of inflammation or imaging evidence of pericardial inflammation may be helpful [10, 11]. Imaging

Table 9.1 Aetiologies of acute pericarditis in major published series from the late 1970s to 2012

	Permanyer-Miralda (Spain)	Zayas (Spain)	Imazio (Italy)	Reuter[a] (South Africa)	Gouriet (France)
Patients (*n*)	231	100	453	233	933
Years	1977–1983	1991–1993	1996–2004	1995–2001	2007–2012
Geographic area	Western Europe	Western Europe	Western Europe	Africa	Western Europe
Idiopathic	199 (86.0 %)	78 (78.0 %)	377 (83.2 %)	32 (13.7 %)	516 (55.0 %)
Specific aetiology	32 (14.0 %)	22 (22.0 %)	76 (16.8 %)	201 (86.3 %)	417 (46.0 %)
Neoplastic	13 (5.6 %)	7 (7.0 %)	23 (5.1 %)	22 (9.4 %)	85 (8.9 %)
Tuberculosis	9 (3.9 %)	4 (4.0 %)	17 (3.8 %)	161 (69.5 %)	4 (<1 %)
Autoimmune	4 (1.7 %)	3 (3.0 %)	33 (7.3 %)	12 (5.2 %)	197 (21 %)
Purulent	2 (0.9 %)	1 (1.0 %)	3 (0.7 %)	5 (2.1 %)	29 (3.0 %)

[a]Based on pericardial effusions.

In the French study, all hospitalized patients were included from a tertiary referral centre for cardiology and infectious diseases. Patients were recruited from emergency department, cardiology and cardiac surgery departments. On this basis, this is a selected view of hospitalized patients with a possible over-representation of specific aetiologies (e.g. infections and post-cardiac injury syndromes) compared to unselected series including also patients who were not hospitalized [8].

Table 9.2 Definitions and diagnostic criteria for acute pericarditis

Pericarditis	Definition and diagnostic criteria
Acute	Inflammatory pericardial syndrome to be diagnosed with at least 2 of the 4 following criteria: 1. Pericarditic chest pain 2. Pericardial rubs 3. New widespread ST elevation or PR depression on ECG 4. Pericardial effusion (new or worsening) Additional supporting findings: Elevation of markers of inflammation (i.e. C-reactive protein, erythrocyte sedimentation rate and white blood cell count) Evidence of pericardial inflammation by an imaging technique (computed tomography, cardiac magnetic resonance)

evidence of pericardial inflammation may be provided by second level imaging techniques, such as computed tomography (CT; as enhanced pericardial imaging after contrast injection) and cardiac magnetic resonance (CMR; as evidence of oedema on T2-weighted dark blood images and late gadolinium enhancement as evidence of organizing pericarditis and/or fibrosis after injection of gadolinium chelates; see chapter on multimodality imaging of the pericardium).

Major differential diagnoses include acute coronary syndromes with ST-segment elevation and early repolarization (see chapter on the diagnosis of pericardial diseases).

Patients with concomitant myocarditis may present with an elevation of markers of myocardial injury (e.g. especially troponin) [11–13].

9.4   Diagnostic Work-Up and Management

The basic diagnostic work-up of patients with acute pericarditis should include:

1. History and physical examination
2. Markers of inflammation and myocardial lesion
3. ECG
4. Chest x-ray
5. Echocardiography

All these evaluations received a class I indication in 2015 ESC guidelines on pericardial diseases (Recommendations Class I, LOE C) [10].

Specific features at presentation have been identified as associated with an increased risk of complications during follow-up and non-viral aetiologies that may warrant targeted therapies (Table 9.3) [14].

On this basis, a triage of patients with pericarditis is possible after the initial evaluation (Fig. 9.5).

It is not mandatory to search for the aetiology in all patients, especially in countries with a low prevalence of tuberculosis, because of the relatively benign course associated with the common causes of pericarditis, and the relatively low diagnostic yield of diagnostic investigations. The recommended diagnostic work-up is focused on the exclusion of the main causes. of acute pericarditis that may warrant a targeted therapy (e.g. bacterial or other infectious aetiologies, cancer, systemic inflammatory diseases) [10].

As reported in Fig. 9.5, any clinical presentation that may suggest an underlying aetiology (e.g. a systemic inflammatory disease) or with at least one predictor of poor prognosis (major or minor risk factors) warrants hospital admission and aetiology search [4, 14].

On the other hand, patients without these features could be managed as outpatients with empiric anti-inflammatories and short-term follow-up after 1 week to assess the response to treatment.

Table 9.3 Indicators of non-viral aetiologies and complications (high-risk features or red flags in acute pericarditis)

Major
Fever >38 °C
Subacute onset
Large pericardial effusion (>20 mm on echocardiography)
Cardiac tamponade
Lack of response to aspirin or NSAID after at least 1 week of therapy
Minor
Pericarditis associated with myocarditis
Immunodepression or Immunosuppression
Trauma
Oral anticoagulant therapy

Major features have been validated in multivariable analysis on prospective cohort study of patients with acute pericarditis [14]

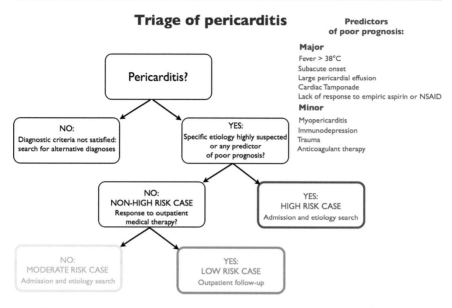

Fig. 9.5 Triage of patients with acute pericarditis. If a patient has one or more prognostic predictor as reported in Table 9.3, he/she is a high-risk patient to be admitted to hospital and aetiology search should be performed. Patients without high-risk features can be managed as outpatient without aetiology search and admission, if there is a good response to empiric anti-inflammatory therapy

Current European guidelines on the management of pericardial diseases recommend hospital admission only for high-risk cases (Class I recommendation, LOE B) and outpatient management for low-risk patients with short-term evaluation at 1 week to assess the response to empiric anti-inflammatory therapies (Class I recommendation, LOE B) [10].

According to clinical presentation, the additional diagnostic work-up should be performed only with a specific clinical suspicion, presence of high-risk features or lack/incomplete response to empiric anti-inflammatory therapy [10].

The detection of the specific viral aetiologies is no more mandatory and cost-effective. Viral serology is expensive, and an extensive serological work-up is not possible in all cases. Moreover the definite diagnosis is based on the demonstration of the virus in pericardial fluid or tissue that would require pericardial fluid and/or tissues analyses and that are often not possible in low-risk cases with mild or no effusions and not cost-effective, since therapy is unchanged and non-specific in immunocompetent patients with uncomplicated course.

A practical clinical approach for the aetiological diagnosis (when really needed) is outlined in Table 9.4 and it is consistent with 2015 ESC guidelines [10].

As a general rule, the main aim of this diagnostic work-up is to exclude the most common and important aetiologies:

1. Bacterial (especially tuberculosis and purulent pericarditis)
2. Cancer (usually secondary pericardial involvement from lung and breast cancer or lymphomas, leukaemias, contiguous cancer, e.g. oesophageal, gastric cancer,

Table 9.4 A practical diagnostic work-up for the evaluation of the aetiology of acute pericarditis in high-risk, complicated cases or when the clinical presentation is highly suggestive of a non-viral aetiology. Modified from 2015 ESC guidelines [10]

Clinical condition	Blood tests	Imaging	Pericardial fluid	Others/red flags
Probable autoimmune condition	Autoantibodies (e.g. ANA, ENA, ANCA) Additional tests according to the specific clinical suspicion	Consider PET (e.g. especially for arteritis or sarcoidosis)	–	Specialist consultation may be useful. Hypereosinophilia (Churg-Strauss), oral and genital aphthae (Behçet); difference in blood pressure between two arms (Takayasu), dry eyes (Sjögren, sarcoidosis) macroglossia (amyloidosis)
Probable TBC	QuantiFERON test	Chest CT scan	*Definite diagnosis:* Acid-fast bacilli staining, mycobacterium cultures PCR for genome *Probable diagnosis:* Adenosine deaminase >40U/l, unstimulated IFN-gamma	Culture and PCR in sputum and other biological fluids Consider pericardial biopsy if other tests are inconclusive
Probable neoplasm	Serum neoplastic markers not specific or sensitive (possible non-specific elevation of CA 125)	Chest and abdomen CT scan, consider PET	*Definite diagnosis:* Cytology (higher volumes of fluid, centrifugation and rapid analysis improve diagnostic yield) *Probable diagnosis:* Tumour markers (e.g. CEA >5 ng/ml or CYFRA 21–1 >100 ng/ml)	Consider pericardial biopsy if other tests are inconclusive

Probable viral infections	No more recommended viral serology, PCR is now preferred to serology (not cost-effective, very limited impact on therapy in most cases) Consider serology for HCV and HIV in specific cases	Genome search with PCR for specific infectious agents, e.g. enteroviruses, adenoviruses, parvovirus B19, HHV-6, CMV, EBV (not cost-effective, very limited impact on therapy in most cases)	Infectious specialist consultation
Probable bacterial infections	Blood cultures before antibiotics if fever >38 °C Serology for *Coxiella burnetii* (if Q-fever is suspected) Serology for *Borrelia* spp. (if Lyme disease is suspected)	Chest CT scan *Definite diagnosis:* Aerobic and anaerobic cultures Glucose	Infectious specialist consultation Consider pericardial biopsy if other tests are inconclusive
Probable autoinflammatory conditions (periodic fevers)	FMF and TRAPS mutations		Possible clues for TRAPS are familiarity and poor response to colchicine
Chronic pericardial effusion	Evaluation of thyroid function (TSH) Evaluation of renal function		Consider appropriate tests for suspected neoplasms and TB
Probable constriction	BNP or pro-NT-BNP if dyspnoea (near-normal findings in pure constriction)	Chest CT scan, CMR, cardiac catheterization	

pleural mesothelioma and melanoma, and rare as primary mainly pericardial mesothelioma)
3. Systemic inflammatory diseases

For bacterial and neoplastic pericarditis the *definite diagnosis* consists of the identification of the aetiological agent in pericardial fluid or tissue, while a *probable diagnosis* is based on the assessment of markers (e.g. ADA, interferon, tumour markers) in pericardial fluid or evidence of the disease elsewhere in patients with concomitant pericarditis and usually moderate to large pericardial effusions. [1, 2]

9.5   Therapy

In the absence of a specific aetiology other than viral (idiopathic), the mainstay of therapy is aspirin or a non-steroidal anti-inflammatory drug (NSAID) provided as attack dose every 8 h to better control symptoms all day (recommendation Class I LOE A) [10]. Colchicine should be added on top of this first choice therapy using weight-adjusted doses and without a loading dose to improve patient compliance (recommendation Class I LOE A) [10, 15–18]. The aims of this anti-inflammatory therapy (Table 9.5) are to:

1. Control chest pain
2. Improve the remission rates at a short-term follow-up (1 week)
3. Prevent recurrences of pericarditis

Corticosteroids should be considered only as a second choice if patients have a history of allergy or hypersensitivity to aspirin/NSAID or are already on corticosteroids for any reason or if there is a specific indication (e.g. systemic inflammatory disease on steroids, pregnancy) [19]. Corticosteroids are not recommended as first

Table 9.5 Empiric anti-inflammatory therapy for acute pericarditis

Drug	Usual dosing	Duration	Tapering
Aspirin	750–1000 mg every 8 h	1–2 weeks	Decrease doses every week, e.g. 750 mg TID for 1 week, then 500 mg TID for 1 week then stop
Ibuprofen	600 mg every 8 h	1–2 weeks	Decrease doses every week, e.g. 600 mg plus 400 mg plus 600 mg for 1 week, then 600 mg plus 400 mg plus 400 mg for 1 week, then 400 mg TID for 1 week then stop
Colchicine	0.5 mg once (<70 kg) or 0.5 mg BID (≥70 kg)	3 months	Not mandatory, alternatively 0.5 mg every other day (<70 kg) or 0.5 mg once (≥70 kg) in the last weeks

Therapy duration is individualized when guided by symptoms and CRP normalization: keep the attack dose and taper only if asymptomatic and CRP is normalized (Class IIa recommendation, LOE B)

line for acute pericarditis (recommendation Class III, LOE C). When prescribed, low to moderate doses of corticosteroids (e.g. prednisone 0.2–0.5 mg/kg/day or equivalent) should be provided for 2–4 weeks followed by gradual tapering (recommendation Class IIa LOE C) [10, 15–18]. Colchicine should be always added on top of this therapy.

If a specific aetiology is identified, a targeted therapy is warranted (see Chap. 10).

The choice of drug should be based on the history of the patient (contraindications, previous efficacy or side effects), the presence of concomitant diseases (favouring aspirin over other NSAIDs when aspirin is already needed as antiplatelet treatment) and physician expertise [20, 21].

Non-pharmacological recommendations include the restriction of physical activity beyond ordinary sedentary life until resolution of symptoms and normalization of CRP for patients not involved in competitive sports and for an arbitrary term of 3 months for athletes [22, 23]. For athletes return to competitive sports is allowed only after symptoms have resolved and diagnostic tests (i.e. CRP, ECG and echocardiogram) have been normalized (recommendation Class IIa LOE C) [10].

9.6 Outcome and Prognosis

In patients with viral or idiopathic pericarditis, the prognosis is relatively good [24–26]. The most common complication is recurrent pericarditis occurring in 20–30 % of cases especially if not treated with colchicine [24]. Colchicine may halve the recurrence rate and should be used starting from the initial attack of pericarditis. Cardiac tamponade as well as constrictive pericarditis is rare (<1 % of cases). The complication risk is related to the aetiology. For instance, the risk of constrictive pericarditis (the most feared complication in the long term) is low after viral/idiopathic pericarditis, intermediate for immune-mediated aetiologies as well as post-cardiac injury syndromes and neoplastic pericarditis (2–5 %) and high for bacterial pericarditis (20–30 %), especially if purulent [24].

> **Key Points**
> - Viral and idiopathic pericarditis are the most common forms of acute pericarditis encountered in clinical practice in developed countries with a low prevalence of tuberculosis.
> - The course of these cases is relatively benign and self-limiting, being recurrences the most common complications.
> - Mainstay of therapy is empiric anti-inflammatory therapy with aspirin or NSAID plus colchicine.
> - Specific features at presentation may suggest the increased risk of complications during follow-up and non-viral aetiologies (e.g. high fever >38 °C [100.4 °F], subacute course with symptoms over several days without a clear-cut acute onset, evidence of large pericardial effusion with diastolic

echo-free space >20 mm, cardiac tamponade, failure to respond within 7 days to aspirin/NSAID, associated myocarditis (myopericarditis), immunodepression, trauma and oral anticoagulant therapy).
- The presence of one or more of these features identifies a potentially high-risk case of acute pericarditis to be admitted. In these cases an aetiology search is mandatory.
- Patients with acute pericarditis and no risk features can be considered as low risk and managed as outpatient. In these cases follow-up is mandatory after 1 week to assess the response to empiric anti-inflammatory therapy.

References

1. Imazio M. Contemporary management of pericardial diseases. Curr Opin Cardiol. 2012;27: 308–17.
2. Imazio M, Gaita F. Diagnosis and treatment of pericarditis. Heart. 2015;101:1159–68.
3. Imazio M, Cecchi E, Demichelis B, Chinaglia A, Ierna S, Demarie D, Ghisio A, Pomari F, Belli R, Trinchero R. Myopericarditis versus viral or idiopathic acute pericarditis. Heart. 2008;94:498–501.
4. Imazio M, Demichelis B, Parrini I, Giuggia M, Cecchi E, Gaschino G, Demarie D, Ghisio A, Trinchero R. Day-hospital treatment of acute pericarditis: a management program for outpatient therapy. J Am Coll Cardiol. 2004;43:1042–6.
5. Imazio M, Spodick DH, Brucato A, Trinchero R, Adler Y. Controversial issues in the management of pericardial diseases. Circulation. 2010;121:916–28.
6. Imazio M, Lazaros G, Picardi E, Vasileiou P, Orlando F, Carraro M, Tsiachris D, Vlachopoulos C, Georgiopoulos G, Tousoulis D, Belli R, Gaita F. Incidence and prognostic significance of new onset atrial fibrillation/flutter in acute pericarditis. Heart. 2015;101:1463–7.
7. Imazio M, Brucato A, Maestroni S, Cumetti D, Dominelli A, Natale G, Trinchero R. Prevalence of C-reactive protein elevation and time course of normalization in acute pericarditis: implications for the diagnosis, therapy, and prognosis of pericarditis. Circulation. 2011;123:1092–7.
8. Gouriet F, Levy PY, Casalta JP, Zandotti C, Collart F, Lepidi H, Cautela J, Bonnet JL, Thuny F, Habib G, Raoult D. Etiology of pericarditis in a prospective cohort of 1162 cases. Am J Med. 2015;128:784.e1–8.
9. Mayosi BM. Contemporary trends in the epidemiology and management of cardiomyopathy and pericarditis in sub-Saharan Africa. Heart. 2007;93:1176–83.
10. Authors/Task Force Members, Adler Y, Charron P, Imazio M, Badano L, Barón-Esquivias G, Bogaert J, Brucato A, Gueret P, Klingel K, Lionis C, Maisch B, Mayosi B, Pavie A, Ristić AD, Sabaté Tenas M, Seferovic P, Swedberg K, Tomkowski W. 2015 ESC Guidelines for the diagnosis and management of pericardial diseases: The Task Force for the Diagnosis and Management of Pericardial Diseases of the European Society of Cardiology (ESC) Endorsed by: The European Association for Cardio-Thoracic Surgery (EACTS). Eur Heart J. 2015;36:2921-64.
11. Imazio M, Gaita F, LeWinter M. Evaluation and Treatment of Pericarditis: A Systematic Review. JAMA. 2015;314:1498–506.
12. Imazio M, Brucato A, Spodick DH, Adler Y. Prognosis of myopericarditis as determined from previously published reports. J Cardiovasc Med (Hagerstown). 2014;15:835–9.
13. Imazio M, Brucato A, Barbieri A, Ferroni F, Maestroni S, Ligabue G, Chinaglia A, Cumetti D, Della Casa G, Bonomi F, Mantovani F, Di Corato P, Lugli R, Faletti R, Leuzzi S, Bonamini R,

Modena MG, Belli R. Good prognosis for pericarditis with and without myocardial involvement: results from a multicenter, prospective cohort study. Circulation. 2013;128:42–9.

14. Imazio M, Cecchi E, Demichelis B, Ierna S, Demarie D, Ghisio A, Pomari F, Coda L, Belli R, Trinchero R. Indicators of poor prognosis of acute pericarditis. Circulation. 2007;115:2739–44.

15. Lotrionte M, Biondi-Zoccai G, Imazio M, Castagno D, Moretti C, Abbate A, Agostoni P, Brucato AL, Di Pasquale P, Raatikka M, Sangiorgi G, Laudito A, Sheiban I, Gaita F. International collaborative systematic review of controlled clinical trials on pharmacologic treatments for acute pericarditis and its recurrences. Am Heart J. 2010;160:662–70.

16. Imazio M, Brucato A, Trinchero R, Spodick D, Adler Y. Individualized therapy for pericarditis. Expert Rev Cardiovasc Ther. 2009;7:965–75.

17. Imazio M, Brucato A, Belli R, Forno D, Ferro S, Trinchero R, Adler Y. Colchicine for the prevention of pericarditis: what we know and what we do not know in 2014 – systematic review and meta-analysis. J Cardiovasc Med (Hagerstown). 2014;15:840–6.

18. Alabed S, Cabello JB, Irving GJ, Qintar M, Burls A. Colchicine for pericarditis. Cochrane Database Syst Rev. 2014;8:CD010652.

19. Imazio M, Brucato A, Cumetti D, Brambilla G, Demichelis B, Ferro S, Maestroni S, Cecchi E, Belli R, Palmieri G, Trinchero R. Corticosteroids for recurrent pericarditis: high versus low doses: a nonrandomized observation. Circulation. 2008;118:667–71.

20. Imazio M, Brucato A, Mayosi BM, Derosa FG, Lestuzzi C, Macor A, Trinchero R, Spodick DH, Adler Y. Medical therapy of pericardial diseases: part I: idiopathic and infectious pericarditis. J Cardiovasc Med (Hagerstown). 2010;11:712–22.

21. Imazio M, Brucato A, Mayosi BM, Derosa FG, Lestuzzi C, Macor A, Trinchero R, Spodick DH, Adler Y. Medical therapy of pericardial diseases: part II: noninfectious pericarditis, pericardial effusion and constrictive pericarditis. J Cardiovasc Med (Hagerstown). 2010;11:785–94.

22. Seidenberg PH, Haynes J. Pericarditis: diagnosis, management, and return to play. Curr Sports Med Rep. 2006;5:74–9.

23. Pelliccia A, Corrado D, Bjørnstad HH, Panhuyzen-Goedkoop N, Urhausen A, Carre F, Anastasakis A, Vanhees L, Arbustini E, Priori S. Recommendations for participation in competitive sport and leisure-time physical activity in individuals with cardiomyopathies, myocarditis and pericarditis. Eur J Cardiovasc Prev Rehabil. 2006;13:876–85.

24. Imazio M, Brucato A, Maestroni S, Cumetti D, Belli R, Trinchero R, Adler Y. Risk of constrictive pericarditis after acute pericarditis. Circulation. 2011;124:1270–5.

25. LeWinter MM. Clinical practice. Acute pericarditis. N Engl J Med. 2014;371:2410–6.

26. Lilly LS. Treatment of acute and recurrent idiopathic pericarditis. Circulation. 2013;127:1723–6.

Acute Pericarditis: Specific Aetiologies (Non-viral, Non-idiopathic)

10

10.1 Bacterial Pericarditis

Bacterial pericarditis is a relatively uncommon cause of pericarditis in adults (no more than 5 % of all unselected cases) if tuberculosis is not endemic [1, 2].

In clinical practice, there are two main forms to consider:

1. Tuberculous pericarditis
2. Purulent pericarditis

Tuberculous Pericarditis

Tuberculous pericarditis represents a secondary localization of tuberculosis having a primary infection in a different organ (generally a previous or concomitant pleura-pulmonary involvement).

The clinical presentation may be acute pericarditis with pericardial effusion, apparently isolated effusion, effusive-constrictive pericarditis or simple constrictive pericarditis.

The diagnosis is important since the mortality rate may be as high as 20–40 % at 6 months after diagnosis and there is a specific treatment to offer [3].

Diagnosis

A *definite diagnosis* of tuberculous pericarditis is based on the demonstration of the presence of tubercle bacilli in the pericardial fluid or tissue. However, a *probable diagnosis* of tuberculous pericarditis can be achieved with evidence of the disease elsewhere (e.g. pulmonary tuberculosis) and concomitant pericarditis, a lympho-cytic pericardial exudate with elevated unstimulated interferon-gamma (uIFN-γ), adenosine deaminase (ADA) or lysozyme levels. An *ex juvantibus diagnosis* is admitted only in countries with a high prevalence of tuberculosis with the demonstration of the response to empiric antituberculous therapy (Table 10.1) [3, 4].

© Springer International Publishing Switzerland 2016
M. Imazio, *Myopericardial Diseases: Diagnosis and Management*,
DOI 10.1007/978-3-319-27156-9_10

Table 10.1 Diagnostic testing for the evaluation of suspected tuberculous pericarditis and pericardial effusion. Modified from 2015 ESC guidelines [3]

1. Initial non-invasive evaluation	Chest x-ray: evidence of pulmonary tuberculosis in 30 % of cases
	Echocardiogram: moderate to large pericardial effusion with frond-like projections, and thick "porridge-like" fluid (suggestive findings but not specific)
	Chest CT scan: pericardial effusion and thickening (>3 mm), typical mediastinal and tracheobronchial lymphadenopathy (>10 mm, hypodense centres, matting), with sparing of hilar lymph nodes
	Culture of sputum, gastric aspirate and/or urine for *Mycobacterium tuberculosis*
	Scalene lymph node biopsy: if pericardial fluid is not accessible and lymphadenopathy present
	Tuberculin skin test/QuantiFERON for TB: limited diagnostic value (only confirm previous contact, valuable in immunocompetent to exclude but not to confirm the diagnosis)
2. Pericardiocentesis	*Therapeutic pericardiocentesis:* cardiac tamponade
	Diagnostic pericardiocentesis: all patients with suspected tuberculous pericarditis and moderate to large pericardial effusions. What to look for in pericardial fluid? 1. Culture for *M. tuberculosis* 2. Quantitative polymerase chain reaction (Xpert MTB/RIF) testing for nucleic acids of *M. tuberculosis* 3. Biochemical tests to distinguish between an exudate and a transudate (fluid and serum protein; fluid and serum LDH) 4. White cell analysis and count, and cytology: a lymphocytic exudate favours tuberculous pericarditis 5. Indirect tests for tuberculous infection: interferon-gamma (IFN-γ), adenosine deaminase (ADA) or lysozyme assay
3. Pericardial biopsy	*Therapeutic" biopsy:* as part of surgical drainage in patients with cardiac tamponade or relapsing effusions after pericardiocentesis or requiring open drainage of pericardial fluid
	Diagnostic biopsy: a diagnostic biopsy is recommended in patients with >3 weeks of illness and without aetiologic (areas with a low prevalence of tuberculosis)
4. Empiric antituberculosis therapy	Trial of empiric antituberculosis chemotherapy is recommended for exudative pericardial effusion, after excluding other causes in areas with a high prevalence of tuberculosis

In *endemic areas with poor resources*, a score has been proposed:

Tuberculous pericarditis is highly suspected if score ≥6 based on the following criteria: fever (1 point), night sweats (1 point), weight loss (2 points), globulin level >40 g/l (3 points) and peripheral leucocyte count <10 × 10⁹/l (3 points).

Medical Therapy

A regimen consisting of rifampicin, isoniazid, pyrazinamide and ethambutol for at least 2 months, followed by isoniazid and rifampicin (total of 6 months of therapy) is effective in treating extrapulmonary tuberculosis. Treatment for 9 months or longer gives no better results and has the disadvantages of increased cost and increased risk of poor compliance [3, 4].

Prognosis

High mortality if untreated. Tuberculous pericarditis has a high risk of evolving in constrictive pericarditis, usually within 6 months in effusive forms. Prompt antibiotic therapy is essential to prevent this progression that occurs from 20 % (especially developed countries) but up to 40 % of cases. Additional treatments that may be useful to prevent constriction include (1) intrapericardial urokinase and (2) adjunctive prednisolone for 6 weeks which may halve this complication (to be avoided in HIV-infected patients since it may increase the risk of HIV-associated malignancies) [5].

Pericardiectomy is recommended if the patient's condition is not improving or is deteriorating after 4–8 weeks of antituberculosis therapy (Recommendation class I, LOE C) [3].

Purulent Pericarditis

In developed countries, nowadays, purulent pericarditis is rare, less than 1 % of cases, and generally manifested as a serious febrile disease (fever >38 °C) with moderate to large pericardial effusions. If purulent pericarditis is suspected, urgent pericardiocentesis is mandatory for diagnosis and therapy. Blood cultures should be performed in any patients with fever >38 °C and pericarditis with or without pericardial effusion [6, 7].

Pericardial fluid is usually purulent, with low pericardial glucose and raised pericardial fluid white cell count with a high proportion of neutrophils. Fluid should be sent for bacterial, fungal and tuberculous studies.

Medical Therapy

Intravenous antimicrobial therapy should be started empirically until microbiological results are available. Pericardial drainage is crucial. Purulent effusions are often heavily loculated and likely to re-accumulate rapidly. Intrapericardial thrombolysis is a possible treatment for cases with loculated effusions in order to achieve an adequate drainage before resorting to surgery. Subxiphoid pericardiostomy and rinsing of the pericardial cavity should be considered [3, 6, 7].

Prognosis

High mortality if untreated. Purulent pericarditis has a high risk of evolving towards constrictive pericarditis [1–3].

10.2 Pericarditis in Renal Failure

Pericardial diseases in renal failure have become less common than in the past but should be considered in the differential diagnoses for pericarditis and pericardial effusion.

There are three main presentations of pericarditis in renal failure: (1) uremic pericarditis, occurring before renal replacement therapy or within 8 weeks from its initiation and related to retention of toxic metabolites; (2) dialysis pericarditis, occurring on dialysis (usually ≥8 weeks after its initiation); and (3) "constrictive pericarditis", only rarely [3, 8–10].

Typical features of these forms of pericarditis include:

1. Chest pain is less frequent (one third of patients are asymptomatic).
2. ECG changes are usually absent since myocardial involvement is absent.
3. Pericardial effusion is often bloody because of the uremic coagulopathy.

Intensive dialysis should be considered in uremic pericarditis; when patients with adequate dialysis develop pericarditis, intensifying dialysis should be considered. Pericardiocentesis may be considered in patients not responding to dialysis. An additional presentation of patients with chronic renal failure is simple pericardial effusion, usually chronic and related to continuous volume overload [8–10].

10.3   Pericardial Involvement in Systemic Autoimmune and Autoinflammatory Diseases

Systemic inflammatory diseases (especially systemic lupus erythematosus, Sjögren syndrome, rheumatoid arthritis, scleroderma, systemic vasculitides, Behçet syndrome, sarcoidosis, and inflammatory bowel diseases) are common causes of pericarditis or "apparently" isolated pericardial effusion. Up to 10 % of patients with pericarditis (often recurrent) have a known systemic inflammatory disease, but rarely pericarditis/pericardial effusion may be the first manifestation of the systemic disease. Usually the degree of pericardial involvement is related with the activity of the systemic disease. Moreover concomitant myocarditis may be present as well, since they are also causes of myocardial inflammatory involvement [11].

A specific subgroup of these patients, especially children, may be affected by *periodic fevers or autoinflammatory diseases*. Periodic fevers are genetic disorders characterized by mutations of genes involved in the regulation of the inflammatory response, without involvement of specific T cells or autoantibodies. The most common autoinflammatory syndromes include Familial Mediterranean Fever (FMF), in which serositis episodes last only 1–3 days, and tumour necrosis factor receptor-associated periodic syndrome (TRAPS), in which the episodes last weeks. Mutations associated with these disorders are rare in recurrent pericarditis. A positive family history for pericarditis or periodic fevers, a poor response to colchicine and the need for immunosuppressive agents are clues to the possible presence of an auto-inflammatory disease. Genetic testing is required for the definite diagnosis [1, 2].

Medical Therapy

The main anti-inflammatory therapy is unchanged. Specific diseases may require corticosteroids or a combination of additional drugs. Management requires a multi-disciplinary approach for diagnosis, therapy and follow-up involving rheumatologists, clinical immunology experts, as well as other involved specialists (e.g. gastroenterologist for inflammatory bowel diseases or experts in pulmonary medicine for sarcoidosis).

For periodic fevers, anti-IL1 (e.g. anakinra) or anti-TNF agents may be considered [1, 2].

10.4   Post-cardiac Injury Syndromes

The term post-cardiac injury syndromes (PCIS) include a group of inflammatory pericardial syndromes (post-myocardial infarction pericarditis, post-pericardiotomy syndrome (PPS) and post-traumatic pericarditis). Such syndromes are presumed to have an autoimmune pathogenesis triggered by an initial damage to pericardial and/or pleural tissues, caused by either myocardial necrosis (late post-myocardial infarction pericarditis or Dressler syndrome), surgical trauma (post-pericardiotomy syndrome (PPS)), accidental thoracic trauma (traumatic pericarditis) or iatrogenic trauma with or without bleeding (pericarditis after invasive cardiac interventions) (Fig. 10.1) [12].

The immune-mediated pathogenesis is supported by a latent period generally of few weeks till the appearance of first manifestations and the response to anti-inflammatory drugs (NSAIDs, corticosteroids, colchicine) with possible recurrences. Pericardial bleeding and pleural incision are triggers for the syndrome. Some forms, such as Dressler syndrome, have become rare with early reperfusion therapy of myocardial infarction; however, it may occur especially in case of even minor bleeding into the pericardium. Post-cardiac injury syndromes are emerging causes of pericarditis in developed countries because of the aging of the population and expansion of interventional techniques (e.g. percutaneous coronary intervention, pacemaker implantation, ablation of arrhythmias).

Definition and Diagnostic Criteria

According to proposed diagnostic criteria for the PPS, the diagnosis of a post-cardiac injury syndrome (PCIS) may be reached after a cardiac injury through the following clinical criteria: (1) fever without alternative causes, (2) pericarditic or pleuritic chest pain, (3) pericardial or pleural rubs, (4) evidence of pericardial and/or (5) pleural effusion with elevated CRP. At least 2 of 5 criteria should be fulfilled [3, 12].

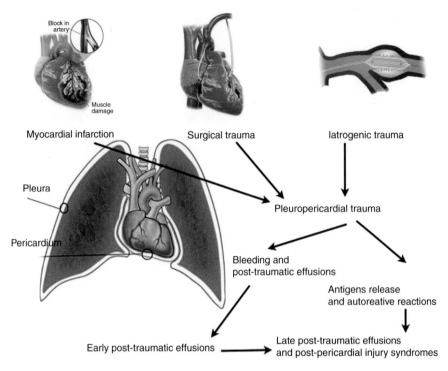

Fig. 10.1 Pathogenesis of post-cardiac injury syndromes, emerging cause of pericardial diseases in developed countries (up to 25 % of cases in last series) due to population ageing and widespread use of percutaneous cardiovascular interventions (see text for explanation)

Specific definitions apply to post-myocardial infarction pericarditis. Two main forms can be recognized:

1. *Early post-infarction pericarditis* usually occurs soon after the AMI and is transient. This complication is rare in the primary percutaneous coronary intervention (PCI) era and is especially related to late reperfusion or failed coronary reperfusion.
2. *Late post-AMI pericarditis (Dressler syndrome)* is rare (<1 %) in the era of primary PCI and may reflect a larger size of AMI and/or late reperfusion.

Medical Therapy

Treatment of post-cardiac injury syndromes is essentially based on empiric anti-inflammatory therapy plus colchicine as outlined for viral or idiopathic pericarditis [3, 12].

Prognosis

The prognosis of the PPS is generally good. Long-term follow-up is warranted since the development of constrictive pericarditis has been reported in about 3 % of cases [13].

10.5   Neoplastic Pericarditis

Neoplastic pericardial involvement is manifested by pericarditis or simple pericardial effusion (usually moderate to large, cardiac tamponade) related to metastatic lymphatic involvement (especially for lung cancer) or haematogenous spread (especially for breast cancer). In addition also lymphomas, leukaemias and melanoma may affect the pericardium, as well as cancer of contiguous organs (e.g. oesophageal cancer). Only rarely neoplastic disease is primary (usually pericardial mesothelioma) [1–3].

Neoplastic pericardial disease may be manifested as pericarditis, pericardial effusion, effusive constrictive pericarditis or constrictive pericarditis. Masses may be diagnosed by imaging techniques.

The definite diagnosis is based on the confirmation of the malignant infiltration within the pericardium by cytology or pericardial biopsy [3, 14]. A probable diagnosis may be achieved by the detection of tumour markers in pericardial fluid (e.g. CEA, CYFRA 21-1, NSE, CA-19-9, CA- 72-4, SCC, GATA3 and VEGF), although none of the tumour markers has been proven to be accurate enough for distinguishing malignant from benign effusions [3]. Evidence of malignant disease elsewhere and concomitant pericarditis or pericardial effusion is also suggestive, although in almost 2/3 of the patients with documented malignancy, pericardial effusion is caused by non-malignant diseases, e.g. radiation pericarditis, other therapies or opportunistic infections [3].

Medical Therapy

The management of these patients require a multidisciplinary approach with oncologists, radiotherapists as well as other subspecialty experts.

General principles of treatment include:

1. Therapeutic and diagnostic pericardiocentesis for the treatment of cardiac tamponade and as diagnostic tool for moderate to large pericardial effusions that are suspected to be of neoplastic aetiology.
2. Systemic antineoplastic treatment as baseline therapy.
3. Pericardial drainage is recommended in all patients with large effusions because of the high recurrence rate (>40–50 %). Additional interventions for recurrent effusions may include pericardiotomy, pericardial window creation and percutaneous balloon pericardiotomy (all techniques are palliative and aimed at improving the quality of life of patients with a poor short-term outcome).
4. Intrapericardial instillation of cytostatic/sclerosing agents to prevent recurrences.
5. Intrapericardial treatment should be tailored to the type of the tumour (e.g. cisplatin is efficacious in lung cancer, thiotepa in breast cancer).
6. Radiation therapy is very effective in controlling malignant pericardial effusion in patients with radiosensitive tumours such as lymphomas and leukaemias.

In clinical practice, management is often palliative at late stages with advanced disease, and it is aimed only at the relief of symptoms rather than treatment of the underlying disease, taking into account the prognosis and the overall quality of life of the patients [3, 14].

10.6 Radiation Pericarditis

Prior chest radiation is an important cause of pericardial disease [15]. Radiation therapy may affect not only the pericardium but also the myocardium, heart valves, coronary arteries and all mediastinal structures inducing fibrosis. Most cases are secondary to radiation therapy for Hodgkin lymphoma or breast or lung cancer, and serious radiation-induced pericardial disease was most often due to radiation therapy of Hodgkin lymphoma. Nowadays lower doses and modern radiation therapy (shielding and dose calculation) have reduced the complications: radiation pericarditis is now dropped from 20 to 2.5 % of cases [3, 15].

Radiation can induce an early disease with pericarditis with or without effusion and a late disease with constrictive pericarditis after 2–20 years and not necessarily preceded by pericarditis. This late disease may affect a variable number of patients (4–20 % of patients) and appears to be dose dependent and related to the presence of late pericardial effusion in the delayed acute phase. The effusion may be serous or haemorrhagic and has a high probability to develop fibrous adhesions. Therapies are similar to those employed in pericarditis and pericardial effusion [3].

The concomitant possible myocardial damage affects the prognosis since radiation-induced constrictive pericarditis has the worse outcome after pericardiectomy [3, 15].

Key Points
- The most common specific forms of acute pericarditis include bacterial (especially tuberculous pericarditis), neoplastic pericarditis and pericarditis related to a systemic inflammatory disease or post-cardiac injury syndromes.
- The definite demonstration of bacterial and neoplastic aetiology requires the identification of the aetiological agent in pericardial fluid (pericardiocentesis) or tissue (pericardial biopsy).
- Each form has specific treatments that should be provided in order to improve the outcomes.
- All these forms have a higher complication risk, especially including the risk of developing constrictive pericarditis in a long-term follow-up.

References

1. Imazio M, Gaita F, LeWinter M. Evaluation and Treatment of Pericarditis: A Systematic Review. JAMA. 2015;314:1498–506.
2. Imazio M, Gaita F. Diagnosis and treatment of pericarditis. Heart. 2015;101:1159–68.

3. Authors/Task Force Members, Adler Y, Charron P, Imazio M, Badano L, Barón-Esquivias G, Bogaert J, Brucato A, Gueret P, Klingel K, Lionis C, Maisch B, Mayosi B, Pavie A, Ristić AD, Sabaté Tenas M, Seferovic P, Swedberg K, Tomkowski W. 2015 ESC Guidelines for the diagnosis and management of pericardial diseases: The Task Force for the Diagnosis and Management of Pericardial Diseases of the European Society of Cardiology (ESC)Endorsed by: The European Association for Cardio-Thoracic Surgery (EACTS). Eur Heart J. 2015;36:2921–64.
4. Mayosi BM, Burgess LJ, Doubell AF. Tuberculous pericarditis. Circulation. 2005;112: 3608–16.
5. Mayosi BM, Ntsekhe M, Bosch J, Pandie S, Jung H, Gumedze F, Pogue J, Thabane L, Smieja M, Francis V, Joldersma L, Thomas KM, Thomas B, Awotedu AA, Magula NP, Naidoo DP, Damasceno A, Chitsa Banda A, Brown B, Manga P, Kirenga B, Mondo C, Mntla P, Tsitsi JM, Peters F, Essop MR, Russell JBW, Hakim J, Matenga J, Barasa AF, Sani MU, Olunuga T, Ogah O, Ansa V, Aje A, Danbauchi S, Ojji D, Yusuf S. Prednisolone and mycobacterium indicus pranii in tuberculous pericarditis. N Engl J Med. 2014;371:1121–30.
6. Sagrista Sauleda J, Barrabés JA, Permanyer Miralda G, Soler Soler J. Purulent pericarditis: review of a 20-year experience in a general hospital. J Am Coll Cardiol. 1993;22:1661–5.
7. Goodman LJ. Purulent pericarditis. Curr Treat Options Cardiovasc Med. 2000;2:343–50.
8. Alpert MA, Ravenscraft MD. Pericardial involvement in end-stage renal disease. Am J Med Sci. 2003;325:228–36.
9. Gunukula SR, Spodick DH. Pericardial disease in renal patients. Semin Nephrol. 2001;21: 52–6.
10. Banerjee A, Davenport A. Changing patterns of pericardial disease in patients with end-stage renal disease. Hemodial Int. 2006;10:249–55.
11. Imazio M. Pericardial involvement in systemic inflammatory diseases. Heart. 2011;97:1882–92.
12. Imazio M, Hoit BD. Post-cardiac injury syndromes. An emerging cause of pericardial diseases. Int J Cardiol. 2013;168:648–52.
13. Imazio M, Brucato A, Maestroni S, Cumetti D, Belli R, Trinchero R, Adler Y. Risk of constrictive pericarditis after acute pericarditis. Circulation. 2011;124:1270–5.
14. Vaitkus PT, Herrmann HC, LeWinter MM. Treatment of malignant pericardial effusion. JAMA. 1994;272:59–64.
15. Stewart JR, Fajardo LF, Gillette SM, Constine LS. Radiation injury to the heart. Int J Radiat Oncol Biol Phys. 1995;31:1205–11.

Recurrent Pericarditis

11

11.1 Definition

Recurrent pericarditis is one of the most common and troublesome complications of acute pericarditis affecting 20–30 % of patients with a first episode of pericarditis and 20–50 % of those with one or multiple recurrences, especially if not treated with colchicine [1].

A true recurrence occurs when there is a symptom-free interval from the previous episode of pericarditis. A minimal time is required since anti-inflammatory therapy with its tapering may be as long as several weeks. This interval has been arbitrarily defined as 4–6 weeks. In the absence of this symptom-free interval, the term "incessant pericarditis" is proposed rather than "recurrent pericarditis", since incessant pericarditis is characterized by continuous symptoms without remission. The term "chronic" is generally referred, especially for pericardial effusions, to disease processes lasting for >3 months, and "chronic pericarditis" is an arbitrary term used by experts for disease lasting >3 months (Table 11.1). All these definitions are consistent with current European guidelines on the management of pericardial diseases [2].

Table 11.1 Definitions of recurrent, incessant and chronic pericarditis

	Definition
Incessant	Pericarditis lasting for >4–6 weeks but <3 months[a] without remission
Recurrent	Recurrence of pericarditis after a documented first episode of acute pericarditis and a symptom-free interval of 4–6 weeks or longer[b]
Chronic	Pericarditis lasting for >3 months[a]

[a]Arbitrary term defined by experts
[b]Usually recurrences occur within 18–24 months for the index attack

© Springer International Publishing Switzerland 2016
M. Imazio, *Myopericardial Diseases: Diagnosis and Management*,
DOI 10.1007/978-3-319-27156-9_11

11.2 Presentation

The usual complain is the recurrence of "pericarditic chest", very often well recognized by patients with the possible association of other symptoms and signs supporting the diagnosis. However, as a general rule, recurrences are essentially manifested by recurrent pain and other manifestations are milder compared with the initial attack of pericarditis and the disease seems to wean slowly with several episodes that are milder and milder with a longer and longer interval between the episodes till complete disappearance of the disease [3–5].

11.3 Aetiology and Diagnosis

The aetiology of recurrent pericarditis is poorly understood. It is supposed to be immune-mediated in most cases, and this statement is supported by the evidence of non-organ-specific autoantibodies and anti-heart antibodies in patients with recurrences as well as response to corticosteroids and colchicine [5–9].

In addition recurrences may be promoted by an underlying disease (e.g. systemic inflammatory disease, cancer), new or recurrent viral infection (as reported in the Marburg experience in 20–30 % of recurrent pericardial effusions), but especially inappropriate treatment of the previous episode of pericarditis (either for low doses of drugs or too short duration of therapy, or too fast tapering), or missed restriction of physical activities (Table 11.2) [4–9].

The diagnosis of recurrent pericarditis is based on an established evidence of a previous attack of acute pericarditis plus "pericarditic pain" and another objective evidence of activity of pericardial inflammatory disease (e.g. pericardial rubs, ECG changes, new or worsening pericardial effusion, elevation of markers of inflammation or white blood cell count). In atypical or doubtful cases, the evidence of pericardial inflammation by an imaging technique is helpful (e.g. pericardial contrast enhancement on CT or evidence of oedema and delayed enhancement on CMR) (Table 11.3) [2, 3].

Table 11.2 Common causes of recurrent pericarditis

Cause	Frequency
Idiopathic	>60–70 %
Infectious (e.g. especially viral)	20–30 %
Systemic inflammatory diseases and pericardial injury syndromes	5–10 %
Autoinflammatory diseases	5–10 %[a]
Neoplastic pericardial diseases	5–10 %
Inadequate treatment of the first or subsequent attack of pericarditis	Unknown[b]

[a]Higher frequency should be suspected especially in children
[b]Inadequate treatment according to doses, duration and tapering and may include the lack of an adequate time of restriction of physical activities

Table 11.3 Diagnostic criteria for incessant, recurrent and chronic pericarditis

Incessant pericarditis is pericarditis lasting for >4–6 weeks but <3 months[a] without remission
Recurrent pericarditis is defined with:
1. A documented first attack of acute pericarditis
2. A symptom-free interval of 4–6 weeks or longer
3. Evidence of subsequent recurrence of pericarditis documented by recurrent pain compatible with pericarditis and one or more of the following signs:
A pericardial friction rub
Changes on electrocardiography
Echocardiographic evidence of new or worsening pericardial effusion
Elevation in the white-cell count, erythrocyte sedimentation rate or C-reactive protein (CRP) level
Chronic pericarditis is pericarditis lasting for >3 months[a]

[a]3 months is an arbitrary time interval defined by experts and reflect the usual resolution of an acute attack of pericarditis within this time interval; recurrences usually occur within 18–24 months, but a precise upper limit of time has not been established

11.4   Diagnostic Work-Up and Management

In patients with recurrences, the diagnostic evaluation is essentially based on (1) confirmation of the diagnosis (according to previously stated diagnostic criteria), (2) evaluation of possible risk factors for complications or non-viral aetiology (e.g. especially moderate to large pericardial effusions or worsening pericardial effusions, cardiac tamponade, incomplete or lacking response to anti-inflammatory therapy), and (3) exclusion of potential specific aetiologies that were missed in the evaluation of the first attacks or previous recurrences for those with multiple recurrences [1–5].

The same high-risk features or red flags presented for acute pericarditis should be considered in patients with recurrent pericarditis. If there are no risk factors and no clues or suspicion of a missed aetiology, there is no reason to repeat aetiological diagnostic tests for each recurrence [2].

11.5   Therapy

The mainstay of therapy for recurrences is physical restriction as non-pharmacological measure till symptom resolution and C-reactive protein normalization and anti-inflammatory therapy based on aspirin or NSAID plus colchicine as first choice as for acute pericarditis (Table 11.4) [7, 10, 11]. Corticosteroids should be considered only after failure of aspirin/NSAID (and more than one of these drugs) [10, 11]. A stepwise approach may be considered: aspirin and NSAID plus colchicine first, then if the patient is still not responding or has additional recurrences, corticosteroids plus colchicine [12–14]. If additional therapy is necessary, a triple therapy may be considered with aspirin or an NSAID plus corticosteroid plus

Table 11.4 Common therapeutic options for recurrent pericarditis

Therapy	Dosing	Duration[a]	Tapering	Monitoring	LOE
Aspirin[b]	750–1000 mg 3 times daily	1–2 weeks	Weekly in 3–4 weeks	Needed	A
Ibuprofen[b]	600 mg 3 times daily	1–2 weeks	Weekly in 3–4 weeks	Needed	A
Indomethacin	50 mg 3 times daily	1–2 weeks	Weekly in 3–4 weeks	Needed	B
Colchicine[b]	0.5 once (<70 kg or chronic kidney disease) or 0.5 mg twice daily	6 months	May be considered	Needed	A
Prednisone	0.2–0.5 mg/kg/day	2–4 weeks	Several months	Needed	B
Azathioprine	Starting with 1 mg/kg day then gradually increased to 2–3 mg/kg/day	Several months	Several months	Needed	C
IVIG	400–500 mg iv daily for 5 days	5 days	Not required	Needed	C
Anakinra	1–2 mg/kg/day up to 100 mg/day in adults	Several months	To be determined	Needed	C
Pericardiectomy	n.a.	n.a	n.a	Needed	C

Monitoring is essentially based on the assessment of blood count, creatinine, creatine kinase (CK), transaminases, C-reactive protein and echocardiography
IVIG IV Immunoglobulins, *n.a.* not applicable, *LOE A* data derived from multiple randomized clinical trials or meta-analyses, *LOE B* data derived from a single randomized clinical trial or large non-randomized studies (in this review, a study with at least made of 100 patients is considered "large"), and *LOE C* consensus of opinion of the experts and/or small studies, retrospective studies and registries
[a]Therapy duration as initial dosing
[b]Aspirin and ibuprofen are common first-level treatments for the first episode of pericarditis (acute pericarditis) associated with colchicine for 3 months

colchicine. In patient on steroids, it is critical to use low to moderate doses (e.g. prednisone 0.2–0.5 mg/day or equivalent) for 4 weeks then slowly tapering after symptom resolution and normalization of C-reactive protein (Table 11.5) [10]. In case of recurrence of symptoms during steroid tapering, which is very common at doses below 15 mg/day of prednisone or equivalent, do not increase again the corticosteroid but try to control the disease increasing or reinstituting aspirin or an NSAID plus colchicine (Fig. 11.1).

Triple therapy for recurrent pericardial pain is similar to multi-drug therapy for angina, where symptom control is achieved by a combination of different drugs [2, 10].

Table 11.5 Tapering of corticosteroids in recurrent pericarditis

Prednisone dose[a]	Starting dose 0.25–0.50 mg/kg/day[a]	Tapering[b]
Prednisone daily dose	>50 mg	10 mg/day every 1–2 weeks
	50–25 mg	5–10 mg/day every 1–2 weeks
	25–15 mg	2.5 mg/day every 2–4 weeks
	<15 mg	1.25–2.5 mg/day every 2–6 weeks

[a]Avoid higher doses except for special cases, and only for a few days, with rapid tapering to 25 mg/day. Prednisone 25 mg is equivalent to methylprednisolone 20 mg
[b]Every decrease in prednisone dose should be done only if the patient is asymptomatic and C-reactive protein is normal, particularly for doses <25 mg/day
Calcium intake (supplement plus oral intake) 1200–1500 mg/day and vitamin D supplementation 800–1000 IU/day should be offered to all patients receiving glucocorticoids. Moreover, bisphosphonates are recommended to prevent bone loss in all men ≥50 years and postmenopausal women in whom long-term treatment with glucocorticoids is initiated at a dose ≥5.0–7.5 mg/day of prednisone or equivalent

Fig. 11.1 A stepwise approach on how to manage recurrences during corticosteroids tapering

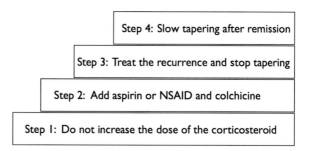

How to manage corticosteroid therapy in case of recurrences during tapering in 4 steps

Step 4: Slow tapering after remission

Step 3: Treat the recurrence and stop tapering

Step 2: Add aspirin or NSAID and colchicine

Step 1: Do not increase the dose of the corticosteroid

Additional therapeutic options to be considered after failure of triple anti-inflammatory therapy include azathioprine, human intravenous immunoglobulins (IVIG) and biological agents (the most common in clinical practice is anakinra) [2, 15–18].

The main mechanism of action of these drugs has been outlined in the chapter on medical therapy of pericardial diseases and it is summarized in Fig. 11.2. A stepwise approach for medical therapy of recurrent pericarditis is reported in Fig. 11.3.

After failure of all options of medical therapy or for those patients who do not tolerate medical therapy or have serious adverse events related to medical therapy, the last possible option is the surgical removal of the pericardium. Total or radical pericardiectomy is recommended in these cases in experienced centres on this surgery [19].

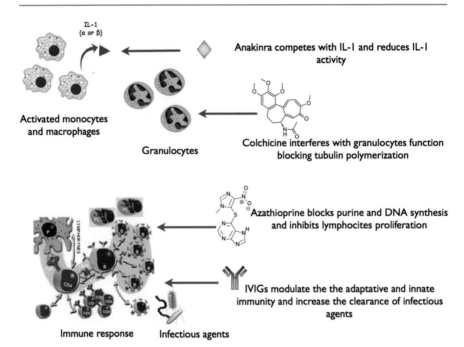

Fig. 11.2 Mechanism of action of emerging new treatments for recurrent pericarditis (e.g. anakinra, colchicine, azathioprine and IVIG)

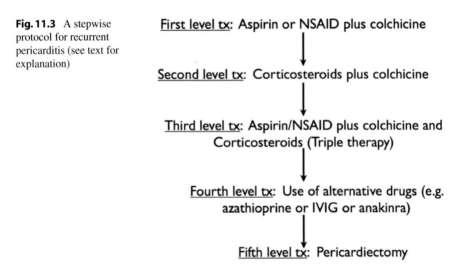

Fig. 11.3 A stepwise protocol for recurrent pericarditis (see text for explanation)

11.6   Outcomes and Prognosis

The overall prognosis of idiopathic recurrent pericarditis (the most common type of recurrence occurring in clinical practice) is good. Despite a possible impairment of the quality of life for a limited time of few years (usually 1–2 years) with several recurrences, there is no risk of increased mortality or chronic evolution. In these patients (idiopathic recurrent pericarditis) constrictive pericarditis has been never described or published in the literature. The risk of constriction is related to the aetiology and not the number of recurrences. In the absence of a missed aetiology, also the risk of cardiac tamponade is very low in idiopathic recurrent pericarditis [20, 21].

Key Points
- Recurrent pericarditis is the most troublesome complication following acute pericarditis and occurring in 20–50 % of patients.
- Most cases of recurrent pericarditis are idiopathic and the pathogenesis is presumed to be immune-mediated or autoinflammatory.
- The mainstay of the therapy of recurrent pericarditis is anti-inflammatory therapy by high doses of aspirin or a NSAID (generally ibuprofen or indomethacin) plus colchicine.
- Second-line drugs are corticosteroids to be used at low to moderate doses (e.g. prednisone 0.2–0.5 mg/kg/day or equivalent) with colchicine till symptom resolution and CRP normalization with a slow tapering and may be combined to aspirin or NSAID plus colchicine in more difficult to treat cases.
- Additional options for patients with multiple failures (≥3) of conventional anti-inflammatory therapies include azathioprine or IVIG or anakinra; these drugs may be added to NSAIDs, colchicine and corticosteroids, if tolerated, in an attempt to obtain remission and withdrawal of corticosteroids.
- Pericardiectomy is the last therapeutic option for patients with true refractory recurrent pericarditis after failure of multiple attempts of medical therapy.
- The prognosis of idiopathic recurrent pericarditis is generally good with the risk of chronic evolution towards constrictive pericarditis related to the aetiology and not the number of recurrences.

References

1. Imazio M, Spodick DH, Brucato A, Trinchero R, Adler Y. Controversial issues in the management of pericardial diseases. Circulation. 2010;121:916–28.
2. Authors/Task Force Members, Adler Y, Charron P, Imazio M, Badano L, Barón-Esquivias G, Bogaert J, Brucato A, Gueret P, Klingel K, Lionis C, Maisch B, Mayosi B, Pavie A, Ristić AD, Sabaté Tenas M, Seferovic P, Swedberg K, Tomkowski W. 2015 ESC Guidelines for the diagnosis and management of pericardial diseases: The Task Force for the Diagnosis and Management of Pericardial Diseases of the European Society of Cardiology (ESC) Endorsed by: The European Association for Cardio-Thoracic Surgery (EACTS). Eur Heart J. 2015;36(42):2921–64.
3. Imazio M, Brucato A, Derosa FG, Lestuzzi C, Bombana E, Scipione F, Leuzzi S, Cecchi E, Trinchero R, Adler Y. Aetiological diagnosis in acute and recurrent pericarditis: when and how. J Cardiovasc Med (Hagerstown). 2009;10:217–30.
4. Soler-Soler J, Sagristà-Sauleda J, Permanyer-Miralda G. Relapsing pericarditis. Heart. 2004; 90:1364–8.

 5. Imazio M, Trinchero R, Shabetai R. Pathogenesis, management, and prevention of recurrent pericarditis. J Cardiovasc Med (Hagerstown). 2007;8:404–10.
 6. Maestroni S, Di Corato PR, Cumetti D, Chiara DB, Ghidoni S, Prisacaru L, Cantarini L, Imazio M, Penco S, Pedrotti P, Caforio AL, Doria A, Brucato A. Recurrent pericarditis: auto-immune or autoinflammatory? Autoimmun Rev. 2012;12:60–5.
 7. Imazio M. Idiopathic recurrent pericarditis as an immune-mediated disease: current insights into pathogenesis and emerging treatment options. Expert Rev Clin Immunol. 2014;10:1487–92.
 8. Imazio M, Brucato A, Doria A, Brambilla G, Ghirardello A, Romito A, Natale G, Palmieri G, Trinchero R, Adler Y. Antinuclear antibodies in recurrent idiopathic pericarditis: prevalence and clinical significance. Int J Cardiol. 2009;136:289–93.
 9. Caforio AL, Brucato A, Doria A, Brambilla G, Angelini A, Ghirardello A, Bottaro S, Tona F, Betterle C, Daliento L, Thiene G, Iliceto S. Anti-heart and anti-intercalated disk autoantibodies: evidence for autoimmunity in idiopathic recurrent acute pericarditis. Heart. 2010;96:779–84.
10. Imazio M, Adler Y. Treatment with aspirin, NSAID, corticosteroids, and colchicine in acute and recurrent pericarditis. Heart Fail Rev. 2013;18:355–60.
11. Imazio M, Lazaros G, Brucato A, Gaita F. Recurrent pericarditis: new and emerging therapeutic options. Nat Rev Cardiol. 2015 Aug 11. doi: 10.1038/nrcardio.2015.115. [Epub ahead of print].
12. Imazio M, Bobbio M, Cecchi E, Demarie D, Pomari F, Moratti M, Ghisio A, Belli R, Trinchero R. Colchicine as first-choice therapy for recurrent pericarditis: results of the CORE (COlchicine for REcurrent pericarditis) trial. Arch Intern Med. 2005;165:1987–91.
13. Imazio M, Brucato A, Cemin R, Ferrua S, Belli R, Maestroni S, Trinchero R, Spodick DH, Adler Y, CORP (COlchicine for Recurrent Pericarditis) Investigators. Colchicine for recurrent pericarditis (CORP): a randomized trial. Ann Intern Med. 2011;155:409–14.
14. Imazio M, Belli R, Brucato A, Cemin R, Ferrua S, Beqaraj F, Demarie D, Ferro S, Forno D, Maestroni S, Cumetti D, Varbella F, Trinchero R, Spodick DH, Adler Y. Efficacy and safety of colchicine for treatment of multiple recurrences of pericarditis (CORP-2): a multicentre, double-blind, placebo-controlled, randomised trial. Lancet. 2014;S0140–6736:62709–9.
15. Vianello F, Cinetto F, Cavraro M, Battisti A, Castelli M, Imbergamo S, Marcolongo R. Azathioprine in isolated recurrent pericarditis: a single centre experience. Int J Cardiol. 2011;147:477–8.
16. Imazio M, Lazaros G, Brucato A, Picardi E, Vasileiou P, Carraro M, Tousoulis D, Belli R, Gaita F. Intravenous human immunoglobulin for refractory recurrent pericarditis. A systematic review of all published cases. J Cardiovasc Med (Hagerstown). 2015 Jun 18. [Epub ahead of print].
17. Lazaros G, Vasileiou P, Koutsianas C, Antonatou K, Stefanadis C, Pectasides D, Vassilopoulos D. Anakinra for the management of resistant idiopathic recurrent pericarditis. Initial experience in 10 adult cases. Ann Rheum Dis. 2014;73:2215–7.
18. Lazaros G, Imazio M, Brucato A, Picardi E, Vassilopoulos D, Vasileiou P, Tousouis D, Gaita F. Anakinra: an emerging option for refractory idiopathic recurrent pericarditis. A systematic review of published evidence. J Cardiovasc Med (Hagerstown). 2015 Jun 18. [Epub ahead of print].
19. Khandaker MH, Schaff HV, Greason KL, Anavekar NS, Espinosa RE, Hayes SN, Nishimura RA, Oh JK. Pericardiectomy vs medical management in patients with relapsing pericarditis. Mayo Clin Proc. 2012;87:1062–70.
20. Brucato A, Brambilla G, Moreo A, Alberti A, Munforti C, Ghirardello A, Doria A, Shynar Y, Livneh A, Adler Y, Shoenfeld Y, Mauri F, Palmieri G, Spodick DH. Long-term outcomes in difficult-to-treat patients with recurrent pericarditis. Am J Cardiol. 2006;98:267–71.
21. Imazio M, Brucato A, Adler Y, Brambilla G, Artom G, Cecchi E, Palmieri G, Trinchero R. Prognosis of idiopathic recurrent pericarditis as determined from previously published reports. Am J Cardiol. 2007;100:1026–8.

Pericarditis Associated with Myocardial Involvement (Myopericarditis/Perimyocarditis)

12

12.1 Definitions

Pericarditis and myocarditis share common aetiological agents (e.g. viruses and also systemic inflammatory diseases). In clinical practice coexistence and overlapping of pericarditis and myocarditis may occur ranging from forms with pure pericarditis, prevalent pericarditis (myopericarditis), prevalent myocarditis (perimyocarditis) to pure myocarditis (Fig. 12.1) [1–3]. In an attempt to provide a clinically useful definition of mixed inflammatory syndromes, the following definitions were proposed [1–4].

Myopericarditis is an inflammatory myopericardial syndrome with prevalent pericarditis with normal biventricular function or without worsening of a previously known ventricular dysfunction. The management and therapy follow the recommendations for pericarditis.

Perimyocarditis is an inflammatory myopericardial syndrome with prevalent myocarditis with evidence of new or worsening ventricular dysfunction. The management and therapy follows the recommendations for myocarditis.

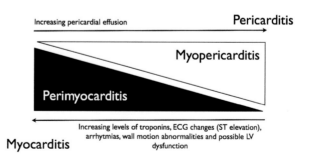

Fig. 12.1 The spectrum of myopericardial syndromes ranging from pure myocarditis to pure pericarditis through intermediate forms (perimyocarditis and myopericarditis)

© Springer International Publishing Switzerland 2016
M. Imazio, *Myopericardial Diseases: Diagnosis and Management*,
DOI 10.1007/978-3-319-27156-9_12

12.2   Presentation

The usual presentation of myopericardial inflammatory syndromes is "pericarditic" chest pain during or following a flu-like syndrome or gastroenteritis, typically in a young male (Table 12.1) [1–3].

In clinical practice, troponin elevation is detected at the initial evaluation at the emergency department [3–6]. Pericardial rubs may be present in forms with prevalent pericarditis. The ECG usually shows widespread ST-segment elevation with possible atypical features and evolution (e.g. localized changes, T wave inversion before ST-segment normalization as in acute coronary syndromes) (Fig. 12.2). Cardiac arrhythmias may be detected usually as premature beats either supraventricular or ventricular. Atrial fibrillation may also occur, while other ventricular arrhythmias are more common in patients with pure myocarditis [3–6].

Patients with myopericarditis, which is pericarditis with mild myocarditis involvement, represent the vast majority of cases encountered in clinical practice. The usual presentation with chest pain may mimic an acute coronary syndrome, which is the main differential diagnosis. On the contrary patients with perimyocarditis may complain a pseudo-infarctual presentation, as well as heart failure or arrhythmic presentation, reflecting the degree of myocardial involvement [1–5].

12.3   Aetiology and Diagnosis

There are three main aetiological categories: idiopathic, infectious and immune mediated (Table 12.2). As mentioned, pericarditis and myocarditis share similar aetiological agents. This aetiological background provides the explanation for overlapping syndromes, although it is not clear why subjects develop pericarditis, myocarditis, mixed forms or no clinical manifestations, despite similar exposition to the same aetiological agent. Unknown genetic and immunological factors probably play a significant role, as well as hormonal factors, since myocardial involvement is more prominent in paediatric cases, as well as young adult males. Limited clinical data on the causes of myopericarditis suggest that viral infections are among the

Table 12.1 Clinical signs and symptoms of myopericarditis

Symptom/sign	Reported frequency
Chest pain	Common
Fever	Common
Fatigue	Frequent
Dyspnoea	Sometimes
Decreased exercise capacity	Frequent
Pericardial rubs	Up to 1/3
ST-segment elevation	>70 %
Cardiac arrhythmias	>50 %
Pericardial effusion	<1/3

most common causes in developed countries. The most frequent viruses encountered in Western Europe and North America include Coxsackieviruses (especially Coxsackie B), Adenoviruses, Cytomegalovirus (CMV), Epstein-Barr Virus (EBV), Influenza virus, Hepatitis A and C virus, Varicella Zoster Virus (VZV) and Parvovirus B19. Fulminant cases have been described in paediatric and adult cases during the pandemic 2009 (H1N1) influenza A, but especially in forms with predominant myocardial involvement, which should be probably more correctly described as myocarditis or perimyocarditis cases, instead of myopericarditis cases [2].

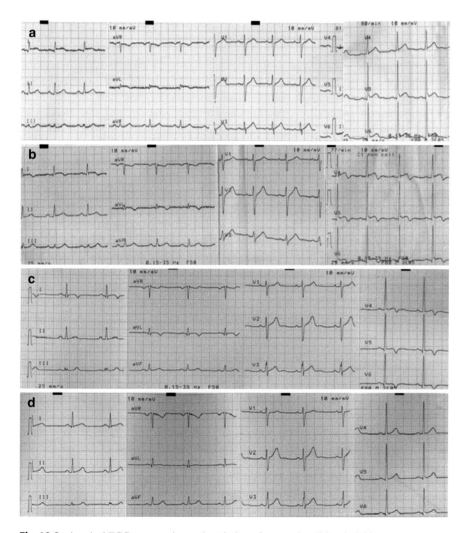

Fig. 12.2 Atypical ECG presentation and evolution of myopericarditis mimicking an acute coronary syndrome with localized ECG changes and T wave inversion before normalization of ST segment. The patient was a 34-year-old male with myopericarditis after a flu-like syndrome (Reproduced with permission from [1])

Table 12.2 Aetiology of myopericarditis and perimyocarditis

Idiopathic
Infectious
Viral (Coxsackie, adenoviruses, herpes viruses, especially CMV, EBV, VZV, influenza, hepatitis A and C, parvovirus B19)
Bacterial (tuberculosis, *Campylobacter jejuni*, *Neisseria meningitides*, *Chlamydophila*)
Other (rare)
Immune-mediated
Systemic inflammatory diseases (giant cell arteritis, systemic lupus erythematosus, adult-onset still disease)
Inflammatory bowel diseases
Vaccine-related (smallpox, diphtheria, tetanus, polio)
Drug-related (5-fluorouracil, phenytoin, clozapine, mesalazine)

Cardiotropic viruses can cause pericardial and myocardial inflammation via direct cytolytic or cytotoxic effects. Viral-induced myocyte damage may lead to the release of intracellular proteins that trigger immunopathic responses in the presence of a predisposing genetic background. Similar mechanisms may play a role in other causes of myopericarditis, such as connective tissue diseases, inflammatory bowel diseases, radiation-induced and drug-induced disease. Among bacterial causes, tuberculosis is probably the most important cause all over the world, because of the high number of cases in developing countries, especially in the setting of HIV co-infection. Increasing reports have been published for *Campylobacter jejuni* as a complication of an acute diarrheal illness and *Shigella*. Pericardial involvement is rare but possible in meningococcal disease and has been described for *Neisseria meningitides* serotypes C, B, W 135, also including cases with myopericarditis. Myopericardial involvement is rare but possible also in infections related to *Chlamydophila pneumoniae*. There is also growing evidence that streptococcal recurrent sore throats, as well as other cases with acute tonsillitis, may be complicated by myopericarditis. Although rare, other bacterial community-acquired pneumonia may be complicated by myopericardial involvement [1, 2].

Myopericarditis is not uncommon in patients with immune-mediated diseases and has been reported in cases with vasculitis, especially giant cell arteritis, systemic lupus erythematosus, adult-onset Still disease, inflammatory bowel diseases especially with recurrent forms and among those exposed to vaccines or certain drugs (i.e. antineoplastic drugs such as 5-fluorouracil, phenytoin, antipsychotic drugs such as clozapine, and mesalazine) [1, 2].

Vaccine-associated myopericarditis has received a special emphasis in the recent years due to the US Federal government campaign to vaccinate military personnel and civilians against smallpox to counter a possible bioterrorism attack and has been described either in military personnel or less frequently in sporadic cases in civilians. Autoimmune reactions following vaccination are rare complications occurring in predisposed individuals and including Guillain-Barrè syndrome after swine influenza vaccine, immune thrombocytopenic purpura after measles/mumps/rubella vaccine and more recently myopericarditis after smallpox vaccination. Molecular mimicry or bystander activation mechanism has been involved. Rarely

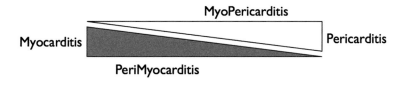

	Pericarditis	MyoPericarditis	PeriMyocarditis
Criteria for pericarditis	+	+	+
Troponin Elevation	negative	usually elevated	usually elevated
EF/WMSI	normal	normal	reduced

Fig. 12.3 Diagnostic features of pericarditis vs. myopericarditis and perimyocarditis. *EF* ejection fraction, *WMSI* wall motion score index. WMSI is abnormal in patients with perimyocarditis. (Reproduced with permission from [9])

myopericarditis has been reported also after other vaccinations (i.e. diphtheria, tetanus and polio) [1, 2].

The diagnosis of *myopericarditis* can clinically be established if patients with definite criteria for acute pericarditis show elevated biomarkers of myocardial injury (troponin I or T, creatine kinase-MB fraction) without newly developed focal or diffuse impairment of left ventricular function in echocardiography or CMR (Fig. 12.3).

On the other hand, evidence of new-onset focal or diffuse reduction of left ventricular function in patients with elevated myocardial biomarkers and clinical criteria for acute pericarditis suggests predominant myocarditis with pericardial involvement (*perimyocarditis*) [1–3].

12.4   Diagnostic Work-Up and Management

Definite confirmation of the presence of myocarditis will require endomyocardial biopsy (EMB) according to Myocardial and Pericardial Diseases WG position statement [7]. However, the benign prognosis of patients with suspected concomitant myocardial involvement in predominant pericarditis (myopericarditis), with absent or mild left ventricular dysfunction, and no symptoms of heart failure does not clinically require endomyocardial biopsy [1–3, 8–10].

In cases of pericarditis with suspected associated myocarditis, coronary angiography (according to clinical presentation and risk factor assessment) is recommended in order to rule out acute coronary syndromes. CMR is recommended for the confirmation of myocardial involvement and to rule out ischaemic myocardial necrosis in the absence of significant coronary disease: this has clinical and therapeutic implications (Fig. 12.4) [1–3].

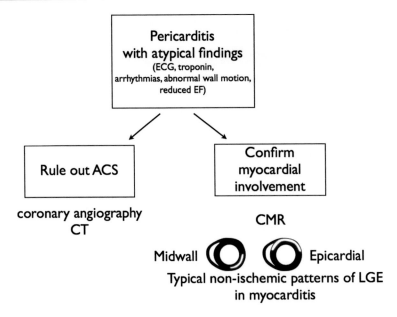

Fig. 12.4 Suggested diagnostic work-up in clinical practice. *LGE* late-gadolinium enhancement

Hospitalization is recommended for diagnosis and monitoring in patients with myocardial involvement and differential diagnosis, especially with acute coronary syndromes (Class recommendation I, LOE C) [4].

A typical pattern of myocardial involvement is documented by LGE with mid-wall, but especially epicardial enhancement. The inferolateral segments are especially involved in most cases.

Current European guidelines recommend coronary angiography (according to clinical presentation and risk factor assessment) in order to rule out acute coronary syndromes (Class recommendation I, LOE C) as well as CMR for the non-invasive confirmation of myocardial inflammatory involvement (Class recommendation I, LOE C) [3].

12.5   Therapy

In the setting of myopericarditis, management is similar to that recommended for pericarditis. Empirical anti-inflammatory therapies (i.e. aspirin 500–1000 mg TID) or NSAIDs (especially ibuprofen 1200–2400 mg/day, or indomethacin 75–150 mg/day) are usually prescribed to control chest pain, while corticosteroids are prescribed as a second choice in cases of contraindication, intolerance or failure of aspirin/NSAIDs [1–5]. In the setting of myopericarditis, some authors recommend reducing dosages, as compared to those adopted for pure pericarditis, because in animal models of myocarditis, NSAIDs have been shown to be non-efficacious and may enhance inflammation, increasing mortality [11]. However, the application of these findings from animal models to humans may be questionable. In addition, there are insufficient data to recommend the use of colchicine, which is a well-established adjunctive treatment for acute and recurrent pericarditis.

Non-pharmacological measures are recommended with exercise restriction beyond normal sedentary activities for 6 months both in athletes and non-athletes (Class recommendation I, LOE C) [4]. For those requiring to be readmitted to competitive sports, a normalization of ECG and echocardiography is required, and exercise testing is usually performed before readmission.

The rationale for this recommendation, essentially based on experts' opinion, is the observation of cases with sudden cardiac death in military forces after strenuous exertion and also in male athletes without prodromal symptoms, who were confirmed to have myocarditis on autopsy [12, 13].

12.6   Outcomes and Prognosis

The great majority of available data, which are however limited to a short–middle-term follow-up, show an overall good prognosis in patients with myopericarditis (i.e. with preserved LV function), despite initial troponin elevation [3, 8–10].

Different considerations may apply for those with perimyocarditis and ventricular dysfunction. For these patients, the same considerations for myocarditis should apply [7].

Several observational series have demonstrated no evolution to heart failure or mortality in patients with myopericarditis [3, 8–10]. The significance of persistent late gadolinium enhancement during follow-up is still unknown. This enhancement is considered expression of fibrosis and it is unclear if it may predispose the patient to any additional risk of arrhythmias or development of heart failure or evolution towards a cardiomyopathy in a long-term follow-up.

Key Points
- Pericarditis and myopericarditis share common aetiological agents and may overlap in inflammatory myopericardial syndromes.
- Myopericarditis is characterized by prevalent pericarditis usually with mild degree of myocarditis, preserved LV function, troponin elevation at presentation.
- The diagnosis is confirmed after exclusion of an ischaemic origin of the presentation by CMR. Coronary angiography may be necessary in cases with a presentation that may mimic an acute coronary syndrome with ST-segment elevation.
- The management follows that outlined for pericarditis, although lower doses of anti-inflammatory drugs are provided aiming at symptoms control, and a longer time of exercise restriction is recommended for both athletes and non-athletes (6 months).
- The prognosis of myopericarditis is benign with no documented excess of mortality or evolution towards a cardiomyopathy or heart failure in short–middle-term follow-up.

References

1. Imazio M, Trinchero R. Myopericarditis: etiology, management, and prognosis. Int J Cardiol. 2008;127:17–26.
2. Imazio M, Cooper LT. Management of myopericarditis. Expert Rev Cardiovasc Ther. 2013; 11:193–201.
3. Imazio M, Brucato A, Barbieri A, Ferroni F, Maestroni S, Ligabue G, Chinaglia A, Cumetti D, Della Casa G, Bonomi F, Mantovani F, Di Corato P, Lugli R, Faletti R, Leuzzi S, Bonamini R, Modena MG, Belli R. Good prognosis for pericarditis with and without myocardial involvement: results from a multicenter, prospective cohort study. Circulation. 2013;128:42–9.
4. Authors/Task Force Members, Adler Y, Charron P, Imazio M, Badano L, Barón-Esquivias G, Bogaert J, Brucato A, Gueret P, Klingel K, Lionis C, Maisch B, Mayosi B, Pavie A, Ristić AD, Sabaté Tenas M, Seferovic P, Swedberg K, Tomkowski W. 2015 ESC Guidelines for the diagnosis and management of pericardial diseases: The Task Force for the Diagnosis and Management of Pericardial Diseases of the European Society of Cardiology (ESC) Endorsed by: The European Association for Cardio-Thoracic Surgery (EACTS). Eur Heart J. 2015;36:2921–64.
5. Imazio M, Cecchi E, Demichelis B, Chinaglia A, Ierna S, Demarie D, Ghisio A, Pomari F, Belli R, Trinchero R. Myopericarditis versus viral or idiopathic acute pericarditis. Heart. 2008;94:498–501.
6. Imazio M, Cecchi E, Demichelis B, Ierna S, Demarie D, Ghisio A, Pomari F, Coda L, Belli R, Trinchero R. Indicators of poor prognosis of acute pericarditis. Circulation. 2007;115:2739–44.
7. Caforio AL, Pankuweit S, Arbustini E, Basso C, Gimeno-Blanes J, Felix SB, Fu M, Heliö T, Heymans S, Jahns R, Klingel K, Linhart A, Maisch B, McKenna W, Mogensen J, Pinto YM, Ristic A, Schultheiss HP, Seggewiss H, Tavazzi L, Thiene G, Yilmaz A, Charron P, Elliott PM, European Society of Cardiology Working Group on Myocardial and Pericardial Diseases. Current state of knowledge on aetiology, diagnosis, management, and therapy of myocarditis: a position statement of the European Society of Cardiology Working Group on Myocardial and Pericardial Diseases. Eur Heart J. 2013;34:2636–48.
8. Buiatti A, Merlo M, Pinamonti B, De Biasio M, Bussani R, Sinagra G. Clinical presentation and long-term follow-up of perimyocarditis. J Cardiovasc Med (Hagerstown). 2013;14:235–41.
9. Imazio M. Pericarditis with troponin elevation: is it true pericarditis and a reason for concern? J Cardiovasc Med (Hagerstown). 2014;15:73–7.
10. Imazio M, Brucato A, Spodick DH, Adler Y. Prognosis of myopericarditis as determined from previously published reports. J Cardiovasc Med (Hagerstown). 2014;15:835–9.
11. Khatib R, Reyes MP, Smith F, et al. Enhancement of coxsackievirus B4 virulence by indomethacin. J Lab Clin Med. 1990;116:116–20.
12. Seidenberg PH, Haynes J. Pericarditis: diagnosis, management, and return to play. Curr Sports Med Rep. 2006;5:74–9.
13. Pelliccia A, Corrado D, Bjørnstad HH, Panhuyzen-Goedkoop N, Urhausen A, Carre F, Anastasakis A, Vanhees L, Arbustini E, Priori S. Recommendations for participation in competitive sport and leisure-time physical activity in individuals with cardiomyopathies, myocarditis and pericarditis. Eur J Cardiovasc Prev Rehabil. 2006;13:876–85.

Pericardial Effusion

13

13.1 Definition

An apparently "isolated" pericardial effusion without pericarditis is another common pericardial syndrome that can be encountered in clinical practice. In physiologic condition, the pericardial space contains 10–50 mL of plasma ultrafiltrate (pericardial fluid) that lubricates the pericardial layers allowing cardiac chamber movements without attrition with the surrounding mediastinal structures [1].

An increased production, usually stimulated by an inflammatory process, or a reduced absorption (e.g. lymphatic obstruction by metastatic spread by lung cancer or pulmonary hypertension or increased filling pressure in heart failure), may be responsible for an increase of the amount of pericardial effusion that starts accumulating posteriorly and inferiorly according to gravity forces (thus a mild effusion is located in inferolateral position and close to the right atrium in four chamber view in transthoracic echocardiography with the patient supine on his/her left side), then as circumferential (moderate to large pericardial effusions) (Fig. 13.1). Thus a pericardial effusion can be defined as an abnormal accumulation of pericardial fluid that can be visualized by echocardiography (the first echocardiographic sign of very mild effusion is systo-diastolic separation on M-mode recordings, while a simple systolic separation may be considered physiologic) (Fig. 13.2) [1, 2].

A common semiquantitative assessment is performed measuring the largest telediastolic echo-free space in different echocardiographic views, including standard and off-axis views. If the size of the effusion is <10 mm, the pericardial effusion is mild; if between 10 and 20 mm, it is moderate; and if >20 mm, the effusion is large (Fig. 13.3) [1–4].

Pericardial effusions can be classified according to the onset (acute, subacute, chronic), the size (usually according to semiquantitative assessment), distribution (loculated and circumferential) and its composition (transudate, exudates, blood, air, etc.).

A practical classification of pericardial effusions is reported in Table 13.1.

© Springer International Publishing Switzerland 2016
M. Imazio, *Myopericardial Diseases: Diagnosis and Management*,
DOI 10.1007/978-3-319-27156-9_13

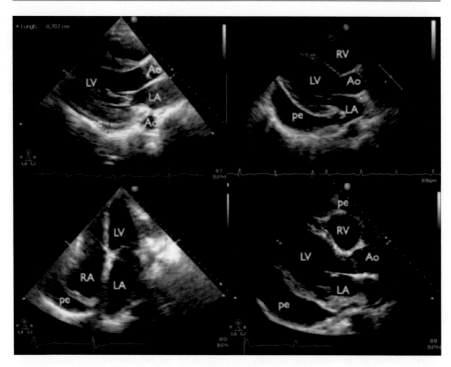

Fig. 13.1 Pericardial effusion (*pe*) of different size on echocardiography. Panel (*images on the left*) a mild effusion that can be seen close to the right atrium (since cardiac chamber with the lowest pressure) and the inferolateral wall of the left ventricle. Panel (*images on the right*) A moderate and large pericardial effusion that is circumferential. *LV* left ventricle, *LA* left atrium, *Ao* aorta, *RV* right ventricle (Reproduced with permission from Imazio and Adler [1])

Fig. 13.2 M-mode recording on echocardiography showing a physiologic systolic separation of pericardial layers. *PW* posterior wall, *PE* pericardial effusion

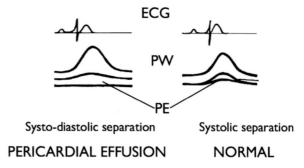

13.2   Presentation

An isolated pericardial effusion may be asymptomatic or has symptoms related to the underlying disease or related to the effusion itself, if moderate to large. Moreover, a pericardial effusion may be an isolated process, but often (50–60 % of cases), it is associated and related to a systemic or underlying disease [5, 6].

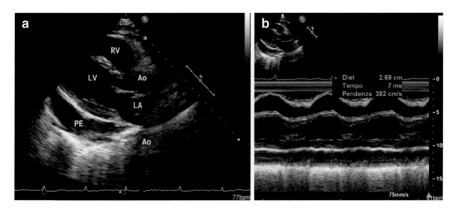

Fig. 13.3 Semiquantitative assessment of pericardial effusion by echocardiography (panel **a**: 2D-echo and panel **b**: M-mode echo): the largest telediastolic echo-free space of 26–27 mm corresponding to a large pericardial effusion. *RV* Right Ventricle, *LV* Left Ventricle, *LA* Left Atrium, *Ao* Aorta, and *PE* Pericardial Effusion

Table 13.1 Classification of pericardial effusions

Onset	Acute
	Subacute
	Chronic (>3 months)
Size	Mild
	Moderate
	Large
Distribution	Circumferential
	Loculated
Composition	Transudate
	Exudate
	Haemopericardium (blood)
	Pneumopericardium (air)
	Chylopericardium (lymphatic liquid)

The speed of its accumulation is critical for the time course of symptoms. Since the pericardium is rather inelastic (as witnessed by a steep relationship between pressure and volume), a rapid accumulating pericardial effusion reaches the limit of pericardial starch very soon with low volumes, while a slowly accumulating fluid reaches the limit of pericardial stretch only for huge volumes as big as 1–2 L without the development of cardiac tamponade [1].

Classical reported symptoms include dyspnoea on exertion progressing to orthopnoea and/or fullness. Additional symptoms may be related to the compressive effect of pericardial effusions on surrounding structures and include nausea (diaphragm), dysphagia (oesophagus), hoarseness (recurrent laryngeal nerve), hiccups (phrenic nerve), cough, weakness, fatigue, anorexia and palpitations (related to the compressive effect of the pericardial fluid or reduced blood pressure) and sinus tachycardia. Additional features (e.g. fever) may be related to the underlying disease (e.g. infectious or systemic inflammatory diseases) more than the pericardial effusion itself [1, 5].

13.3   Aetiology and Diagnosis

The aetiology of pericardial effusion is varied and reflects the potential complexity of the full aetiological spectrum of pericardial diseases including infectious and non-infectious causes.

The most common reported causes include infections (viral, especially tuberculosis that is the most common cause all over the world) [7, 8], cancer (especially lung and breast cancer, lymphomas and leukemias), systemic inflammatory diseases, post-cardiac injury syndromes (emerging cause in developing countries and related to the increased use of invasive cardiovascular interventions and ageing of the population), heart failure, pulmonary hypertension, hypothyroidism and renal failure (Table 13.2) [6, 9–12].

The relative frequency of different causes depends on potential selection biases (geographic area, hospital setting, diagnostic testing). Nevertheless, the majority of cases remain "idiopathic" (about 50 % of cases), that is, without a precise aetiological definition after the diagnostic work-up. In clinical practice, the most common causes to be considered (in the absence of specific clues from the patient) include pericarditis and infectious causes (15–30 %), especially tuberculosis (main cause in developing countries with >60 % of cases), cancer (10–25 %), iatrogenic causes including post-cardiac injury syndromes (15–20 %) and connective tissue disease (5–15 %) [3, 5].

Table 13.2 Aetiologic diagnosis of moderate to large pericardial effusions according to major published series

Feature	Corey et al.	Sagrista-Sauleda et al.	Levy et al.	Reuter et al.	Ma et al.
Patients	57	322	204	233	140
Study years	1993	1990–1996	1998–2002	1995–2001	2007–2009
Country	USA	Spain	France	South Africa	China
Effusion size	>5 mm	>10 mm	NR	NR	Moderate to large[a]
Cardiac tamponade	NR	37	NR	NR	NR
Idiopathic	7	29	48	14	9
Cancer	23	13	15	9	39
Infections	27	2	16	72	29
Connective tissue diseases	12	5	10	5	6
Metabolic	24	6	12	0	0
Iatrogenic	0	16	0	0	9

Data are reported as percentages
NR not reported
[a]All effusions requiring pericardiocentesis

When a pericardial effusion is suspected, the definite diagnosis is simple and relies on transthoracic echocardiography (Class I recommendation, LOE C) [4]. Pericardial effusion has been one of the first applications of the technique, and still nowadays it is essential for its diagnosis.

13.4   Diagnostic Work-Up and Management

After the echocardiographic confirmation of the presence of pericardial effusion, the next steps are reached by the same exam.

It is important to assess:

1. The size (as semiquantitative evaluation since moderate to large effusions are more common in specific aetiologies, such as bacterial and cancer)
2. The haemodynamic importance (presence or not of cardiac tamponade) [13, 14]

Cardiac tamponade and a moderate to large effusion with a clinical suspicion of bacterial or neoplastic aetiology are all indications for pericardiocentesis (Class I recommendation, LOE C) [4]. Cardiac tamponade is especially common in the setting of neoplastic pericardial effusions. Routine diagnostic assessments to be performed on pericardial fluid are listed in Table 13.3.

Since pericarditis is a common cause of pericardial effusion, the presence of possible criteria for the diagnosis (e.g. pericardial rubs, ECG changes) and elevation of markers of inflammation (e.g. C-reactive protein) should be performed (Class I recommendation, LOE C) [4].

Table 13.3 Diagnostic analyses for pericardial fluid

Analysis	Test	Aetiology or feature
General chemistry	Specific gravity > 1015, protein level > 3 g/dl, protein fluid/serum ratio >0.5, LDH >200 mg/dl, fluid/serum ratio >0.6[a]	Exudate
Cytology	Cytology (higher volumes of fluid, centrifugation and rapid analysis improve diagnostic yield)	Cancer
Biomarkers	Tumour markers (i.e. CEA >5 ng/ml or CYFRA 21–1 > 100 ng/ml)	Cancer
	Adenosine deaminase >40U/l, IFN-gamma	TBC
Polymerase chain reaction (PCR)	PCR for specific infectious agents (i.e. TBC)	TBC
Microbiology	Acid-fast bacilli staining, mycobacterium cultures, aerobic and anaerobic cultures	TBC Other bacteria

LDH lactate dehydrogenase, *TBC* tuberculosis
[a]These chemical features have been especially validated for pleural fluid and not pericardial fluid, although generally used also for pericardial effusion

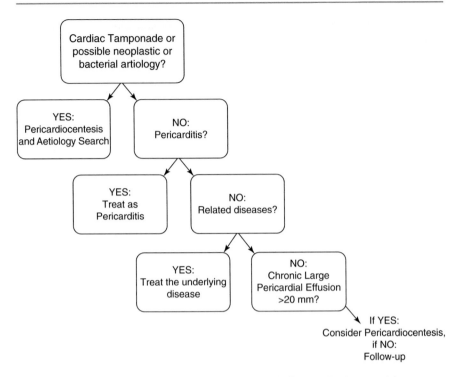

Fig. 13.4 Management algorithm and triage for pericardial effusion of unknown origin

Since up to 60 % of cases of pericardial effusions are related to an underlying disease, it is also important to collect an appropriate history of concomitant diseases and to exclude most important causes (especially cancer, systemic inflammatory diseases, tuberculosis, hypothyroidism and renal failure) [6]. A pericardial effusion may be also related to heart failure and pulmonary hypertension.

On this basis, it is possible to develop a simple basic clinical algorithm for the management of pericardial effusions in clinical practice (Fig. 13.4).

If the patient has cardiac tamponade or a suspected bacterial or neoplastic presentation, admission is recommended for pericardiocentesis and aetiological search. If not, it is important to exclude pericarditis, a diagnosis that is often overlooked in clinical practice. If the patient has signs or symptoms of pericarditis and/or evidence of elevation of C-reactive protein without other causes, the management of the effusion is that of pericarditis. An otherwise unexplained pericardial effusion with a potentially related systemic disease should be managed accordingly. For those cases with a moderate to large pericardial effusion, follow-up is warranted. If the effusion is large (>20 mm) and chronic, there is a potential risk of development of cardiac tamponade during follow-up [15], especially for precipitating causes, such as pericarditis or trauma. The alternative options (pericardiocentesis vs. echocardiographic follow-up) should be clearly explained to the patient, as well as potential benefits and risks of the interventions. The decision is here based on expert and clinical opinion without solid data supporting a specific recommendation and should be taken on an individual basis taking into account the clinical presentation and preferences of the patient, as well as the echocardiographic evolution of the effusion and local expertise.

13.5 Therapy

The therapy of pericardial effusion should be targeted at the aetiology as much as possible (Class I recommendation, LOE C) [4]. Empiric anti-inflammatory therapy (Table 13.4) is recommended for patients with pericardial effusion and evidence of systemic inflammation (e.g. elevation of C-reactive protein). When pericardial effusion is associated with pericarditis, management should follow that of pericarditis [3–5].

In about 50–60 % of cases, the effusion is associated with a known disease, and the essential treatment is that of the underlying disease [3–6].

When a pericardial effusion becomes symptomatic without evidence of inflammation or when empiric anti-inflammatory drugs are not successful, drainage of the effusion should be considered and the size of the effusion is especially large (>20 mm). Pericardiocentesis with prolonged pericardial drainage till <25–30 ml/24 h is recommended to promote adherence of pericardial layers and prevent further accumulation of fluid. If pericardiocentesis is not feasible or fails, alternative surgical options include the creation of a pericardial window either by conventional heart surgery or video-assisted thoracoscopy. Balloon pericardiotomy is an alternative to surgical creation of a pericardial window that has been shown successful especially in the setting

Table 13.4 Empiric anti-inflammatory therapy for inflammatory pericardial effusions

Drug	Attack dose	Treatment length	Level of evidence[a]
Acetylsalicylic acid	750–1000 mg tid	1–2 weeks	B
Ibuprofen	600 mg tid	1–2 weeks	B
Indomethacin	25–50 mg tid	1–2 weeks	C
Prednisone or steroid at equivalent dose	0.2–0.5 mg/kg/day	First episode: 2 weeks Recurrence: 4 weeks	B
Colchicine	0.5 mg bid (>70 kg) 0.5 mg once (<70 kg)	First episode: 3 months Recurrence: 6 months	A A

Tapering may be considered in case of normalization of markers of inflammation and significant response to therapy (symptoms, regression or reduction of pericardial effusion). A low tapering is especially required for corticosteroids (i.e. decrease prednisone 2.5 mg every 2–4 weeks)
tid three times daily, *bid* twice daily
[a]A in case of multiple randomized trials or meta-analysis, B for a single randomized trial or non-randomized studies, C for consensus opinion of experts

of neoplastic pericardial disease as a palliative measure in patients with a limited life expectancy. The technique involves inserting a deflated single catheter or double balloon catheters into the pericardial space using a subxiphoid approach under fluoroscopic or echocardiographic guidance. The last surgical option especially for those with recurrent large symptomatic pericardial effusions or cardiac tamponade is pericardiectomy that should be performed in experienced centre for pericardial surgery. The need of intervention in all cases remains controversial and requires the understanding of the possible benefit/risk ratio (i.e. invasive interventions as a possible trigger of recurrences since induce pericardial bleeding).

Unfortunately there are no proven effective medical therapies to reduce an isolated effusion in the absence of inflammation. NSAID and colchicine and corticosteroids are generally not efficacious.

13.6   Outcomes and Prognosis

The prognosis of pericardial effusion is essentially related to the aetiology, and thus it is important to identify specific aetiology that requires targeted therapies. The size of the effusion is correlated to prognosis, because moderate to large effusions are more common for specific aetiologies such as bacterial, neoplastic or related to a systemic inflammatory disease [3–5].

Large chronic effusions of "idiopathic" aetiology have a progression risk to cardiac tamponade of about 30 % and related to precipitating events (e.g. pericarditis, chest trauma) [15].

Echocardiographic monitoring is recommended especially for moderate to large pericardial effusions. The follow-up of pericardial effusion is mainly based on the evaluation of symptoms, current therapies and the echocardiographic size of the effusion, as well as additional features such as inflammatory markers (i.e. C-reactive protein). New 2015 ESC guidelines recommend the following times [4] that are in agreement with my clinical experience:

– A mild idiopathic effusion (<10 mm) is usually asymptomatic, has a generally good prognosis and does not require specific monitoring.
– A moderate to large effusions (>10 mm) warrant echocardiographic monitoring: every 6 months if moderate and every 3–6 months for large effusions.

A tailored follow-up is warranted also considering the relative stability or evolution of the size (i.e. a worsening effusion may require a closer timing also guided by symptoms).

> **Key Points**
> • Pericardial effusions are especially caused by pericarditis, systemic inflammatory diseases, cancer, post-cardiac injury syndromes, trauma, hypothyroidism and renal failure.

- An overlooked pericarditis should be excluded in all cases.
- If the presentation is with cardiac tamponade or a bacterial or neoplastic aetiology is suspected, there is indication for pericardiocentesis.
- In 50–60 % of cases, pericardial effusion is related to underlying diseases and management should be targeted to them, accordingly.
- If systemic inflammation (e.g. elevation of C-reactive protein) is detected with associated pericardial effusion without alternative causes, an attempt to treat the effusion with empiric anti-inflammatory therapy is warranted.
- The prognosis of the effusion is essentially related to the aetiology and its size.
- Echocardiographic monitoring (every 3–6 months) is warranted in moderate to large pericardial effusions according to the size, time evolution, symptoms and patient preferences.
- The risk of cardiac tamponade is not negligible in those with chronic large "idiopathic" effusions especially because of precipitating events such as pericarditis and chest trauma.

References

1. Imazio M, Adler Y. Management of pericardial effusion. Eur Heart J. 2013;34:1186–97.
2. Permanyer-Miralda G. Acute pericardial disease: approach to the aetiologic diagnosis. Heart. 2004;90:252–4.
3. Imazio M, Brucato A, Mayosi BM, Derosa FG, Lestuzzi C, Macor A, Trinchero R, Spodick DH, Adler Y. Medical therapy of pericardial diseases: part II: noninfectious pericarditis, pericardial effusion and constrictive pericarditis. J Cardiovasc Med (Hagerstown). 2010;11:785–94.
4. Authors/Task Force Members, Adler Y, Charron P, Imazio M, Badano L, Barón-Esquivias G, Bogaert J, Brucato A, Gueret P, Klingel K, Lionis C, Maisch B, Mayosi B, Pavie A, Ristić AD, Sabaté Tenas M, Seferovic P, Swedberg K, Tomkowski W. 2015 ESC Guidelines for the diagnosis and management of pericardial diseases: the task force for the diagnosis and management of pericardial diseases of the European Society of Cardiology (ESC) endorsed by: the European Association for Cardio-Thoracic Surgery (EACTS). Eur Heart J. 2015;36:2921–64.
5. Imazio M, Mayosi BM, Brucato A, Markel G, Trinchero R, Spodick DH, Adler Y. Triage and management of pericardial effusion. J Cardiovasc Med (Hagerstown). 2010;11:928–35.
6. Sagrista-Sauleda J, Merce J, Permanyer-Miralda G, Soler-Soler J. Clinical clues to the causes of large pericardial effusions. Am J Med. 2000;109:95–101.
7. Mayosi BM. Contemporary trends in the epidemiology and management of cardiomyopathy and pericarditis in sub-Saharan Africa. Heart. 2007;93:1176–83.
8. Mayosi BM, Burgess LJ, Doubell AF. Tuberculous pericarditis. Circulation. 2005;112:3608–16.
9. Corey GR, Campbell PT, Trigt V, Kenney RT, O'Connor CM, Sheikh KH, Kisslo JA, Wall TC. Etiology of large pericardial effusions. Am J Med. 1993;95:209–13.
10. Levy PY, Corey R, Berger P, et al. Etiologic diagnosis of 204 pericardial effusions. Medicine (Baltimore). 2003;82:385–91.
11. Reuter H, Burgess LJ, Doubell AF. Epidemiology of pericardial effusions at a large academic hospital in South Africa. Epidemiol Infect. 2005;133:393–9.
12. Ma W, Liu J, Zeng Y, Chen S, Zheng Y, Ye S, Lan L, Liu Q, Weig HJ, Liu Q. Causes of moderate to large pericardial effusion requiring pericardiocentesis in 140 Han Chinese patients. Herz. 2012;37:183–7.

13. Shabetai R. Pericardial effusion: haemodynamic spectrum. Heart. 2004;90:255–6.
14. Spodick DH. Acute cardiac tamponade. N Engl J Med. 2003;349:684–90.
15. Sagristà-Sauleda J, Angel J, Permanyer-Miralda G, Soler Soler J. Long-term follow-up of idiopathic chronic pericardial effusion. N Engl J Med. 1999;341:2054–9.

Cardiac Tamponade

14

14.1 Definition

Cardiac tamponade is the pericardial syndrome occurring when pericardial effusion impairs diastolic filling of the heart till reducing cardiac output and producing signs and symptoms. The impairment of diastolic filling is continuous through the entire diastole. The size of the effusion as well as its distribution may be variable [1, 2].

Since the pericardium is relatively stiff, if a pericardial fluid collects quickly, such as in haemopericardium, the limit of pericardial stretch is reached soon with volumes of 200–300 mL; on the contrary a slowly accumulating pericardial effusion may reach 1–2 L before the development of cardiac tamponade [3, 4]. This pathophysiology explains that cardiac tamponade is a last-drop phenomenon. Thus a small increase of pericardial volume may precipitate the syndrome, and also the aspiration of small amounts of pericardial fluid may greatly improve the clinical condition in urgent pericardiocentesis [5].

Usually pericardial effusions are circumferential, but after trauma or cardiac surgery, they may be loculated and even be responsible for localized compression and the development of cardiac tamponade.

14.2 Presentation

The classical presentation of cardiac tamponade has been described by the thoracic surgeon, Beck in 1935 (Fig. 14.1) [5, 6]. Beck identified a *triad including hypotension, increased jugular venous pressure and a small and quiet heart.*

This triad was classically identified in "surgical tamponade" with acute cardiac tamponade due to intrapericardial haemorrhage because of trauma and myocardial or aortic rupture. The Beck triad may be lacking in patients with "medical tamponade" with slowly accumulating pericardial fluid. Hypotension is absolute or relative. Acute cardiac tamponade is usually associated with low blood pressure (<90 mmHg) but only slightly reduced in subacute and chronic tamponade.

© Springer International Publishing Switzerland 2016   123
M. Imazio, *Myopericardial Diseases: Diagnosis and Management*,
DOI 10.1007/978-3-319-27156-9_14

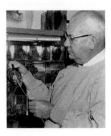

Signs
Classical Beck triad
(Beck 1935)

TWO CARDIAC COMPRESSION TRIADS
CLAUDE S. BECK, M.D.
CLEVELAND

Lesions of the pericardium are generally difficult problems in diagnosis. Auenbrugger, Corvisart and Laennec early recognized these difficulties. Osler not infrequently lamented his failure to recognize a lesion of the pericardium and it would seem that these problems in diagnosis still exist. The chief reason for failure in the diagnosis of pericardial lesions is the fact that the physiologic concept of acute and chronic compression of the heart has not found the place in applied medicine that it deserves. Clinically, almost all of the intrapericardial lesions express themselves, if they express themselves at all, by producing either acute or chronic compression of the heart. Some lesions of the pericardium are entirely silent; they produce no clinical signs whatever and clinical recognition of these silent lesions is not to be expected. However, the important group of lesions—important because treatment is effective produces either acute or chronic compression of the heart. In this respect the intrapericardial lesion producing compression of the heart is exactly similar to the intracranial lesion producing either acute or chronic pressure on the brain. The intrapericardial lesion, like the intracranial lesion, produces clear and distinctive earmarks for recognition. In the case of the heart the earmarks for both acute

- # Hypotension

- # Increasing jugular venous pressure

- # small, quiet heart

J Am Med Assoc. 1935;104:714-716.

Fig. 14.1 The classical Beck triad in patients with acute cardiac tamponade (*J Am Med Assoc* 1935;104:714–716)

Hypertensive patients may have normal to mildly elevated blood pressure concomitant to cardiac tamponade [5, 6].

On physical examination, classical signs include neck vein distention with *elevated jugular venous pressure at bedside examination, pulsus paradoxus* and *diminished heart sounds* on cardiac auscultation. Pulsus paradoxus has been described for the first time by Kussmaul in 1873 as a palpable reduction of radial pulse on inspiration in patients with cardiac tamponade. The so-called paradox was the "waxing and waning" of the peripheral pulse, in contrast to the unvarying strength of the apical cardiac impulse. Pulsus paradoxus is classically defined as an inspiratory reduction of at least 10 mmHg of the systolic blood pressure. It can be easily detected by recording the systolic pressure at which Korotkoff sounds are first audible and the systolic pressure at which they are audible through the whole respiratory cycle (Fig. 14.2) [5, 6].

Pulsus paradoxus is due to exaggerated ventricular interdependence occurring in cardiac tamponade when overall volume of cardiac chambers becomes fixed and any change in the volume of one side of the heart causes the opposite changes in the other side (i.e. inspiratory increase of venous return and right chambers with decreased left chambers volume and reduced systemic blood pressure) (Fig. 14.3). On ECG, the patient usually shows tachycardia, low QRS voltages and electrical alternans. Both ECG signs are non-specific and are considered related to the damping effect of pericardial fluid and swinging heart [5, 6].

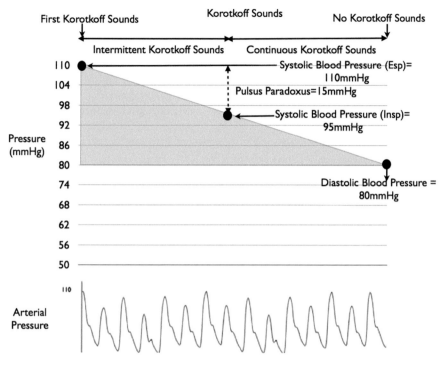

Fig. 14.2 How to measure pulsus paradoxus. Pulsus paradoxus is classically defined as an inspiratory reduction of at least 10 mmHg of the systolic blood pressure (in this case it is 15 mmHg). It can be easily detected by recording the systolic pressure at which Korotkoff sounds are first audible (110 mmHg in this case) and the systolic pressure at which they are audible through the whole respiratory cycle (95 mmHg in this case)

Exaggerated interventricular interdependence in cardiac tamponade (Inspiration)

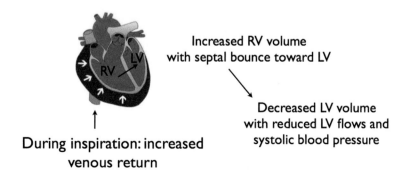

Fig. 14.3 Inspiratory decrease of systolic pressure during inspiration in cardiac tamponade (see text for additional explanation)

14.3   Aetiology and Diagnosis

All the causes of pericardial effusion are also possible causes of cardiac tamponade. In clinical practice the most common aetiologies include cancer, tuberculosis
and purulent infections, trauma, iatrogenic complication of cardiovascular interventions (e.g. ablation of arrhythmias, pacemaker implantation, percutaneous
coronary intervention), acute aortic disease, systemic inflammatory diseases and
renal failure [4, 5].

The diagnosis of cardiac tamponade is a clinical diagnosis based on the combination of a suggestive history and symptoms (typically dyspnoea on exertion progressing to orthopnoea, chest pain and/or fullness) together with elevated jugular venous
pressure at bedside examination, pulsus paradoxus, diminished heart sounds and
often hypotension. The clinical suspicion of cardiac tamponade should be confirmed
by echocardiography. Echocardiography can be performed bedside and in urgent/
emergency situations and demonstrates moderately large or large circumferential
pericardial effusion, signs of right atrial and/or right ventricular compression and
abnormal respiratory variation in right and left ventricular dimensions and in tricuspid and mitral valve flow velocities usually associated with inferior vena cava plethora (Table 14.1 and Fig. 14.4) [3–5].

14.4   Diagnostic Work-Up and Management

The diagnosis of cardiac tamponade identifies a high-risk subject with an
increased risk of complications during follow-up and a high probability of a non-
viral aetiology. The patient should be admitted for therapy and monitoring
[7–10].

The definite therapy is pericardiocentesis that should be performed on an urgent
basis according to clinical presentation.

Table 14.1 Echocardiographic signs of cardiac tamponade

Echocardiographic feature	Sensitivity	Specificity
Large pericardial effusion with swinging heart	n.a.	n.a.
Diastolic collapse of the right atrium (RA)	50–100 %	33–100 %
Duration of diastolic collapse of the RA as ratio on the cardiac cycle length >0.34	>90 %	100 %
Diastolic collapse of the right ventricle	48–100 %	72–100 %
Respiratory changes of the mitral E velocity >25 %, tricuspid E velocity >40 %	n.a.	n.a.
Inferior vena cava plethora (dilatation >20 mm and <50 % reduction of diameter with respiratory phases)	97 %	40 %

n.a. not available

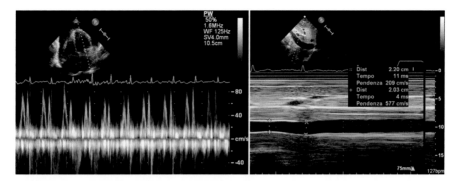

Fig. 14.4 Respiratory changes of mitral E velocity >25 % and inferior vena cava (IVC) plethora (>20 mm with respiratory variations <50 %) in a patient with cardiac tamponade (Reproduced with permission from Imazio and Adler [4])

A triage system (Fig. 14.5) has been proposed by the ESC Working Group on myocardial and pericardial diseases in order to guide the timing of the intervention and the possibility of transfer to a referral centre [5]. However this system is essentially based on expert's opinion and requires additional validation before a recommendation could be done on its routinary implementation in clinical practice.

14.5   Therapy

The treatment of cardiac tamponade is drainage of the pericardial fluid, preferably by needle pericardiocentesis with the use of echocardiographic or fluoroscopic guidance that should be performed without delay in unstable patients. Alternatively drainage is performed by a surgical approach, especially in some situations such as purulent pericarditis or urgent situations with bleeding into the pericardium.

Pericardiocentesis should be performed by experienced operators and carries a variable risk of complications from 4 to 10 % depending on type of monitoring, skills of the operator and setting (emergency vs. urgent vs. elective). Most common complications include arrhythmias, coronary artery or cardiac chamber puncture, haemothorax, pneumothorax, pneumopericardium and hepatic injury [10].

14.6   Outcomes and Prognosis

The prognosis of cardiac tamponade is essentially related to the aetiology. Cardiac tamponade in patients with cancer and metastatic involvement of the pericardium has a bad short-term prognosis since it is a sign of advanced cancer disease; on the contrary, patients with cardiac tamponade and a final diagnosis of idiopathic pericarditis have a generally good long-term prognosis [7–10].

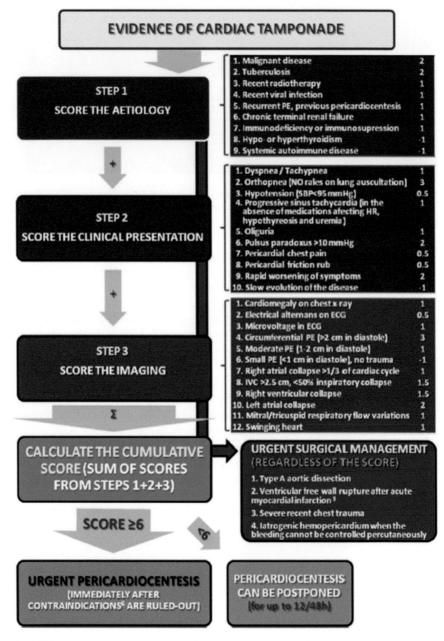

Fig. 14.5 Proposed triage of cardiac tamponade according to the Working Group on myocardial and pericardial diseases of the European Society of Cardiology (ESC) (Reproduced with permission from Ristić et al. [5])

Key Points
- Cardiac tamponade occurs when pericardial effusion compresses the heart and impairs diastolic filling till reduction of the cardiac output.
- Pericardial effusion and cardiac tamponade share common aetiologies.
- The diagnosis of cardiac tamponade is a clinical diagnosis based on suggestive history and clinical presentation with worsening dyspnoea, distended jugular veins, muffled heart sounds and pulsus paradoxus and should be confirmed by echocardiography.
- Cardiac tamponade is a life-threatening syndrome that requires urgent treatment by pericardiocentesis.
- The prognosis of cardiac tamponade is related to the underlying cause.

References

1. Shabetai R. Pericardial effusion: haemodynamic spectrum. Heart. 2004;90:255–6.
2. Spodick DH. Acute cardiac tamponade. N Engl J Med. 2003;349:684–90.
3. Imazio M, Mayosi BM, Brucato A, Markel G, Trinchero R, Spodick DH, Adler Y. Triage and management of pericardial effusion. J Cardiovasc Med (Hagerstown). 2010;11:928–35.
4. Imazio M, Adler Y. Management of pericardial effusion. Eur Heart J. 2013;34:1186–97.
5. Ristić AD, Imazio M, Adler Y, Anastasakis A, Badano LP, Brucato A, Caforio AL, Dubourg O, Elliott P, Gimeno J, Helio T, Klingel K, Linhart A, Maisch B, Mayosi B, Mogensen J, Pinto Y, Seggewiss H, Seferović PM, Tavazzi L, Tomkowski W, Charron P. Triage strategy for urgent management of cardiac tamponade: a position statement of the European Society of Cardiology Working Group on Myocardial and Pericardial Diseases. Eur Heart J. 2014;35:2279–84.
6. Roy CL, Minor MA, Brookhart MA, Choudhry NK. Does this patient with a pericardial effusion have cardiac tamponade? JAMA. 2007;297:1810–8.
7. Imazio M, Cecchi E, Demichelis B, Ierna S, Demarie D, Ghisio A, Pomari F, Coda L, Belli R, Trinchero R. Indicators of poor prognosis of acute pericarditis. Circulation. 2007;115:2739–44.
8. Imazio M, Brucato A, Mayosi BM, Derosa FG, Lestuzzi C, Macor A, Trinchero R, Spodick DH, Adler Y. Medical therapy of pericardial diseases: part II: noninfectious pericarditis, pericardial effusion and constrictive pericarditis. J Cardiovasc Med (Hagerstown). 2010;11:785–94.
9. Permanyer-Miralda G. Acute pericardial disease: approach to the aetiologic diagnosis. Heart. 2004;90:252–4.
10. Authors/Task Force Members, Adler Y, Charron P, Imazio M, Badano L, Barón-Esquivias G, Bogaert J, Brucato A, Gueret P, Klingel K, Lionis C, Maisch B, Mayosi B, Pavie A, Ristić AD, Sabaté Tenas M, Seferovic P, Swedberg K, Tomkowski W. 2015 ESC guidelines for the diagnosis and management of pericardial diseases: the task force for the diagnosis and management of pericardial diseases of the European Society of Cardiology (ESC) endorsed by: the European Association for Cardio-Thoracic Surgery (EACTS). Eur Heart J. 2015;36:2921–64.

Constrictive Pericarditis

15

15.1 Definition

Constrictive pericarditis is a pericardial syndrome where the pericardium becomes relatively rigid and inelastic, may be thickened and calcified or not, and impairs mid to late diastolic filling. Constrictive pericarditis is the final pathway of several different diseases or causes, usually causing pericarditis and pericardial effusion and progressing towards pericardial fibrosis and calcification [1–3].

In constrictive pericarditis, the typical impairment of diastolic filling is mid to late diastolic with a suddenly blocked early diastolic filling causing several signs on physical examination (pericardial knock) and echocardiography (septal notch on M-mode, 2D echo recordings). In addition the fibrotic evolution of the pericardium is responsible for the obliteration of pericardial space with dissociation of intrathoracic pressures from intracardiac pressures as in cardiac tamponade. On this basis, the overall pericardial volume becomes fixed and the increase of one ventricle (e.g. right ventricle during inspiration due to increased venous return) can only occur with the decrease of the other (e.g. left ventricle). This causes and exaggerated interventricular interdependence with inspiratory decrease of the left ventricle volume and flows and contemporary increase right ventricle volume and flow with septal bulging that can be seen on echocardiography [1–3].

15.2 Presentation

The typical presentation of a patient with constrictive pericarditis includes signs and symptoms of right heart failure usually with preserved right and left ventricular function in the absence of previous or concomitant myocardial disease or advanced forms. Patients complain about dyspnoea, fatigue, peripheral oedema, breathlessness, hepatomegaly, pleural effusions, ascites and abdominal swelling. The delay between the initial pericardial inflammation and the

© Springer International Publishing Switzerland 2016
M. Imazio, *Myopericardial Diseases: Diagnosis and Management*,
DOI 10.1007/978-3-319-27156-9_15

onset of constriction is variable and it is possible a direct evolution from subacute/chronic pericarditis to constrictive pericarditis [3]. In specific forms such as in tuberculous pericarditis or effusion, the evolution usually occurs within 3–6 months [3, 4].

In advanced cases, pericardial fibrosis and scarring may extend into the myocardium, thus causing myocardial fibrosis and dysfunction. In specific forms (e.g. radiation pericarditis), the same aetiological agent (radiation) affecting the pericardium also affects the myocardium (as well as valves and coronary arteries), thus causing ventricular dysfunction as well.

15.3   Aetiology and Diagnosis

Constrictive pericarditis is commonly the final evolution of any type of pericarditis and pericardial effusion. The risk of developing such evolution is especially related to the aetiology: low (<1 %) in viral and idiopathic pericarditis, intermediate (2–5 %) in immune-mediated pericarditis and neoplastic pericardial diseases, and high (20–30 %) in bacterial pericarditis, especially purulent pericarditis [5].

There are few contemporary series of constrictive pericarditis reported by tertiary referral centres after pericardiectomy (Stanford, Mayo Clinic, Cleveland Clinic, and Groote Schuur Hospital) (Table 15.1) [6–9].

Table 15.1   Major published series on constrictive pericarditis

Feature	Cameron et al. [6]	Ling et al. [7]	Bertog et al. [8]	Mutyaba et al. [9]
Institution	Stanford University	Mayo Clinic	Cleveland Clinic	Groote Schuur Hospital
Country	USA	USA	USA	South Africa
Years	1970–1985	1985–1995	1977–2000	1990–2012
Patients	95	135	163	121
Cause				
Idiopathic	40 (42 %)	45 (33 %)	75 (46 %)	6 (5 %)
Post-radiation	29 (31 %)	17 (13 %)	15 (9 %)	0 (0 %)
Post-surgery	10 (11 %)	24 (18 %)	60 (37 %)	0 (0 %)
Post-infectious	6 (6 %)	26 (20 %)	7 (4 %)	110 (91 %)[a]
Connective tissue disease	4 (4 %)	10 (7 %)	5 (3 %)	0 (0 %)
Other	6 (6 %)	13 (10 %)	1 (1 %)	5 (4 %)

As for acute pericarditis, most cases are idiopathic in developed countries with a low prevalence of tuberculosis, while tuberculosis is the most important cause in developing countries
[a] 36 patients (29.8 %) had proven tuberculosis, and 74 patients (61.2 %) had presumed tuberculosis

The most common reported causes were idiopathic or viral (42–49 %), post-cardiac surgery (11–37 %), post-radiation therapy (9–31 %), mostly for Hodgkin's disease or breast cancer, connective tissue disorder (3–7 %), post-infectious (tuberculous or purulent pericarditis in 3–6 %) and miscellaneous causes (malignancy, trauma, drug-induced, asbestosis, sarcoidosis, uremic pericarditis in less than 10 %) in developed countries [6–9]. However, tuberculosis is a major cause all over the world, especially because of developing countries, where tuberculosis is endemic [4].

In final stages, when constriction is chronic and permanent, it may be difficult to distinguish the initial cause, since the final picture of fibrosis and scarring on bioptic samples, and the clinical presentation are non-specific [3].

According to 2015 ESC guidelines on the management of pericardial diseases, the diagnosis of constrictive pericarditis is based on the association of signs and symptoms of right heart failure and instrumental evidence of an impaired diagnostic filling due to pericardial constriction by one or more imaging methods including echocardiography, CT, CMR and cardiac catheterization [4]. Although classical and advanced cases show prominent pericardial thickening and calcifications in chronic forms (Figs. 15.1 and 15.2), constriction may also be present with normal pericardial thickness in up to 20 % of cases [10].

The main differential diagnosis is with restrictive cardiomyopathy (Table 15.2). The essential differential features between the two pathological conditions are represented by the affected part of the heart. In "simple" (not advanced or complicated by ventricular dysfunction) constrictive pericarditis, it is the pericardium to be involved and not the myocardium, while in restrictive cardiomyopathy, it is the

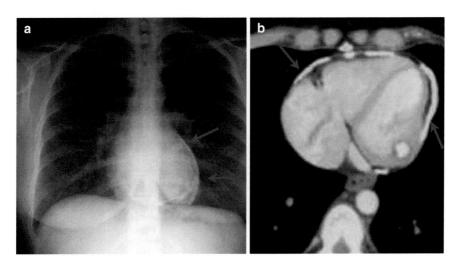

Fig. 15.1 Calcifications may be detected in about one third of cases on chest x-ray (see *arrows* on panel **a**) and are also evaluated on CT scan (see *arrows* on panel **b**) that allows a better study of their extension for surgical planning of pericardiectomy

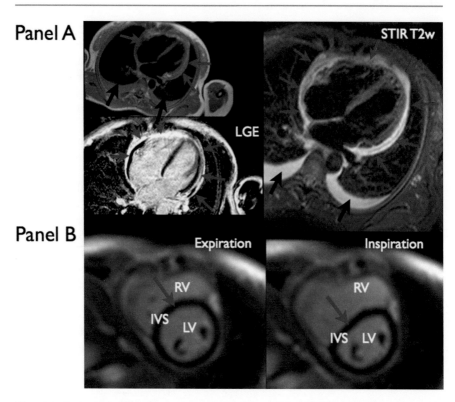

Fig. 15.2 Pericardial thickening with pericardial inflammation on CMR study (see *red arrows* in panel (**a**), pericardial oedema on STIR T2w image and pericardial late gadolinium enhancement, concomitant pleural effusion is marked with *black arrows*). On panel (**b**) it is evident septal bounce (see *red arrows*) due to exaggerated interventricular interdependence by real-time CMR imaging. *LGE* late gadolinium enhancement, *RV* right ventricle, *IVS* interventricular septum, *LV* left ventricle

left ventricle at the myocardial level to be involved. In constrictive pericarditis, this implies that diastolic dysfunction affects the mid-late diastole with dissociation of intrathoracic with intracardiac pressures and essentially preserved myocardial function.

Nowadays non-invasive imaging is sufficient to clarify the diagnostic suspicion in most cases with constrictive pericarditis. Thus, the role of cardiac catheterization is essentially limited to the preoperative assessment of coronary angiography and especially to clarify atypical presentation with discordant data from non-invasive imaging [1, 2, 4, 11, 12].

Exaggerated interventricular interdependence is a main feature of constrictive pericarditis, and Mayo Clinic also proposed a haemodynamic criterion based on this feature, and with a high diagnostic accuracy (the *systolic area index*). The systolic area index (SAI) is defined as the ratio of the RV area (mmHg x s) to the LV area (mmHg x s) in inspiration versus expiration. A SAI>1.1 is diagnostic for constrictive pericarditis [12].

Table 15.2 Constrictive pericarditis vs. restrictive cardiomyopathy: a comparison of main clinical and instrumental findings for the differential diagnosis

Diagnostic evaluation	Constrictive pericarditis	Restrictive cardiomyopathy
Physical findings	Kussmaul sign, pericardial knock	Regurgitant murmur, Kussmaul sign +/−, S3 (advanced)
ECG	Low voltages, non-specific ST/T changes, atrial fibrillation	Low voltages, pseudoinfarction, possible widening of QRS, left-axis deviation, atrial fibrillation
Chest x-ray	Pericardial calcifications (1/3)	No pericardial calcifications
Echocardiography	Septal bounce Pericardial thickening and calcifications	Small left ventricle with large atria, possible increased wall thickness
	Respiratory variation of the mitral peak E velocity of >25 % and variation in the pulmonary venous peak D flow velocity of >20 %	E/A ratio >2, short DT, significant respiratory variations of mitral inflow are absent
	Colour M-mode flow propagation velocity (Vp) >45 cm/s	Colour M-mode flow propagation velocity (Vp) <45 cm/s
	Tissue Doppler: peak e' >8.0 cm/s	Tissue Doppler: peak e' <8.0 cm/s
Cardiac catheterization	"Dip and plateau" or "square root" sign, right ventricular diastolic, and left ventricular diastolic pressures usually equal, ventricular interdependence (i.e. assessed by the systolic area index >1.1)[a]	Marked right ventricular systolic hypertension (>50 mmHg) and left ventricular diastolic pressure exceeds right ventricular diastolic pressure (LVEDP > RVEDP) at rest or during exercise by 5 mmHg or more (RVEDP <1/3 RVSP)
CT/CMR	Pericardial thickness >3–4 mm, pericardial calcifications (CT), ventricular interdependence (real-time cine CMR)	Normal pericardial thickness (<3.0 mm), myocardial involvement by morphology and functional study (CMR)

S3 third sound, *DT* deceleration time, *LVEDP* left ventricular end-diastolic pressure, *RVEDP* right ventricular end-diastolic pressure, *CMR* cardiac magnetic resonance
Kussmaul sign is a paradoxical rise in jugular venous pressure on inspiration
[a]The systolic area index was defined as the ratio of the RV area (mmHg × s) to the LV area (mmHg × s) in inspiration versus expiration

15.4 Diagnostic Work-Up and Management

In a patient with a clinical suspicion of constrictive pericarditis, the diagnosis should be confirmed by echocardiography first (Class I recommendation, LOE C) [4]. Echocardiographic signs of constriction include septal bounce, suspicion of pericardial thickening and calcifications on M-mode and 2D-echocardiography (the assessment of pericardial thickness should be performed by CT or CMR). On Doppler echocardiography, there is evidence of exaggerated interventricular interdependence with respiratory variation of the mitral peak E velocity of >25 % and variation in the pulmonary venous peak D flow velocity of >20 %. On colour M-mode flow propagation velocity (Vp) >45 cm/s (normal in the absence of myocardial involvement). Also tissue Doppler findings should be normal in the absence of myocardial involvement or extensive calcifications (e.g. tissue Doppler: peak e' >8.0 cm/s) [1, 2, 11].

Specific diagnostic echocardiographic criteria for the diagnosis of constrictive pericarditis have been recently proposed by the Mayo Clinic and include septal bounce or ventricular septal shift with either medial $e' > 8$ cm/s or hepatic vein expiratory diastolic reversal ratio>0.78 (sensitivity 87 %, specificity 91 %; specificity may increase to 97 % if all criteria are present with a correspondent decrease of sensitivity to 64 %) [11].

Additional diagnostic findings include non-specific ST/T abnormalities on ECG and atrial fibrillation may be present. Pericardial calcifications are detected by chest x-ray in about one third of cases [13].

CT and CMR are recommended second-level imaging modality (Class I recommendation, LOE C) that allow the quantification of pericardial thickness, although in about 20 % of cases, the pericardium may be not thickened [4, 10].

CT is especially useful for the assessment of calcifications, and it is commonly requested by cardiac surgeons for the planning of pericardiectomy (Fig. 15.1).

CMR allows additional functional study and assessment on cine-real-time imaging of septal bounce and interventricular interdependence (Fig. 15.2). Moreover, the detection of evidence of pericardial inflammation in cases with new-onset constriction may allow to identify potential transient and reversible forms [14–18].

As previously mentioned, cardiac catheterization is indicated when non-invasive diagnostic methods provide discordant or non-conclusive data for the diagnosis (Class I recommendation, LOE C) [4].

15.5   Therapy

Medical therapy has specific indications: (1) to prevent the progression to constriction (e.g. anti-tuberculous antibiotic therapy); (2) to treat pericardial inflammation as a cause of potentially reversible constriction when detected by clinical evidence of pericarditis or pericardial inflammation on CT/CMR; and (3) supportive therapy for heart failure in advanced cases and when surgery is contraindicated or at high risk [3, 4].

The definite therapy of chronic constriction is radical pericardiectomy. Surgical removal of the pericardium has a significant operative mortality ranging from 6 to 12 %. Pericardiectomy must be as complete as possible and should be performed by experienced centres. Surgery should be considered cautiously in patients with advanced disease and in those with radiation-induced constriction, myocardial dysfunction or significant renal dysfunction. Prior radiation therapy is associated with a poor long-term outcome, because it induces myocardial dysfunction as well as pericardial disease. Predictors of poor overall survival are prior radiation, worse renal function, higher pulmonary artery systolic pressure, abnormal left ventricular systolic function, lower serum sodium level and older age [19–22].

Table 15.3 Definitions and therapy of main constrictive pericardial syndromes

Syndrome	Definition	Therapy
Transient constriction (d.d. permanent constrictive pericarditis, restrictive CMP)	Reversible pattern of constriction following spontaneous recovery or medical therapy	A 2–3-month course of empiric anti-inflammatory medical therapy
Effusive-constrictive pericarditis (d.d. cardiac tamponade, constrictive pericarditis)	Failure of the right atrial pressure to fall by 50 % or to a level below 10 mmHg after pericardiocentesis. May be diagnosed also by non-invasive imaging	Pericardiocentesis followed by medical therapy. Surgery for persistent cases
Chronic constriction (d.d. transient constriction, restrictive CMP)	Persistent constriction after 3–6 months	Pericardiectomy, medical therapy for advanced cases or high risk of surgery or mixed forms with myocardial involvement

d.d. differential diagnosis, *CMP* cardiomyopathy

The classical description of chronic permanent constrictive pericarditis has been challenged by specific forms of constrictive syndromes (i.e. transient constriction, effusive-constrictive forms). Definitions, main differential diagnoses and treatment of main constrictive pericardial syndromes are summarized in Table 15.3.

Effusive-constrictive pericarditis deserves a special mention. Effusive-constrictive pericarditis is caused especially by tuberculosis in developing countries. Most cases of effusive-constrictive pericarditis are idiopathic in developed countries, reflecting the frequency of idiopathic pericardial disease in general. Other reported causes include radiation, neoplasia, chemotherapy, infections (especially tuberculosis and purulent forms) and postsurgical pericardial disease. Patients with effusive-constrictive pericarditis have both a fibrotic and scarred pericardium (often with special involvement of the epicardium) plus pericardial effusion. Patients with effusive-constrictive pericarditis usually have clinical features of pericardial effusion or constrictive pericarditis or both. The constrictive physiology is often masked by cardiac tamponade and right atrial pressure is persistently elevated after pericardiocentesis. The classical haemodynamic criterion is the failure of the right atrial pressure to fall by 50 % or to a level below 10 mmHg after pericardiocentesis. Although the traditional diagnosis is made by invasive measurement of right atrial pressure, nowadays, it may be well diagnosed also by non-invasive imaging.

The definite therapy of cases with persistent constriction is pericardiectomy with a special attention to the removal of visceral pericardium that is often involved in this condition [23, 24].

15.6 Outcomes and Prognosis

The outcome of constriction is related to the background conditions (e.g. previous radiation therapy carries a poor prognosis, concomitant renal failure), patient age and especially the presence of concomitant myocardial dysfunction. Survival after

Table 15.4 Child-Pugh score classification for the severity of cirrhosis

Criteria	Points		
	1	2	3
Encephalopathy	None	Grade 1 or 2	Grade 3 or 4
Ascites	None	Mild to moderate (diuretic responsive)	Severe (diuretic refractory)
Bilirubin (mg/dL)	<2	2–3	>3
Albumin (g/dL)	>3.5	2.8–3.5	<2.8
Prothrombin time			
Second prolonged or	<4	4–6	>6
INR	<1.7	1.7–2.3	>2.3

Class A = 5 to 6 points, Class B = 7 to 9 points, Class C = 10 to 15 points
INR international normalized ratio

radical pericardiectomy in patients with scores Child-Pugh B or C (CP score ≥ 7) has been reported to be significantly worse than in patients with CP-A (Table 15.4). In multivariable analysis, a Child-Pugh score of 7 or more, mediastinal irradiation, advanced age and end-stage renal disease identified and increased risk of death after radical pericardiectomy. Child-Pugh scoring system may be helpful for the prediction of mortality after radical pericardiectomy in patients with constrictive pericarditis, who should undergo this surgery [22].

Key Points
- Constrictive pericarditis is the usual final destination of complicated cases of pericarditis/pericardial effusions, especially with a bacterial aetiology.
- In constrictive pericarditis, a fibrotic pericardium impairs diastolic filling in mid to late diastole and dissociates intrathoracic pressures from intracardiac pressures, thus generating an exaggerated interventricular interdependence.
- The clinical picture is that of right heart failure with a preserved ventricular function if cases are not advanced or complicated by concomitant myocardial dysfunction.
- The clinical suspicion should be confirmed by echocardiography and additional non-invasive imaging techniques including CT and CMR.
- Cardiac catheterization is limited to atypical or complex presentation when non-invasive methods are not able to confirm the diagnosis.
- Calcifications can be detected in one third of cases on chest x-ray and are better studied on CT scan. The presence of calcifications is not mandatory for the diagnosis.
- Constriction may occur even with a normal thickness of the pericardium in about 20 % of cases and may be transient if caused by pericardial inflammation.
- The definite therapy of permanent/chronic constriction is radical pericardiectomy to be performed in skilled centres for this surgery.

References

1. Klein AL, Abbara S, Agler DA, Appleton CP, Asher CR, Hoit B, Hung J, Garcia MJ, Kronzon I, Oh JK, Rodriguez ER, Schaff HV, Schoenhagen P, Tan CD, White RD. American Society of Echocardiography clinical recommendations for multimodality cardiovascular imaging of patients with pericardial disease: endorsed by the Society for Cardiovascular Magnetic Resonance and Society of Cardiovascular Computed Tomography. J Am Soc Echocardiogr. 2013;26:965–1012.e15.
2. Cosyns B, Plein S, Nihoyanopoulos P, Smiseth O, Achenbach S, Andrade MJ, Pepi M, Ristic A, Imazio M, Paelinck B, Lancellotti P, On behalf of the European Association of Cardiovascular Imaging (EACVI) and European Society of Cardiology Working Group (ESC WG) on Myocardial and Pericardial diseases. European Association of Cardiovascular Imaging (EACVI) position paper: multimodality imaging in pericardial disease. Eur Heart J Cardiovasc Imaging. 2014;16:12–31.
3. Imazio M, Brucato A, Mayosi BM, Derosa FG, Lestuzzi C, Macor A, Trinchero R, Spodick DH, Adler Y. Medical therapy of pericardial diseases: part II: noninfectious pericarditis, pericardial effusion and constrictive pericarditis. J Cardiovasc Med (Hagerstown). 2010;11:785–94.
4. Authors/Task Force Members, Adler Y, Charron P, Imazio M, Badano L, Barón-Esquivias G, Bogaert J, Brucato A, Gueret P, Klingel K, Lionis C, Maisch B, Mayosi B, Pavie A, Ristić AD, Sabaté Tenas M, Seferovic P, Swedberg K, Tomkowski W. 2015 ESC guidelines for the diagnosis and management of pericardial diseases: the task force for the diagnosis and management of pericardial diseases of the European Society of Cardiology (ESC) endorsed by: the European Association for Cardio-Thoracic Surgery (EACTS). Eur Heart J. 2015;36:2921–64.
5. Imazio M, Brucato A, Maestroni S, Cumetti D, Belli R, Trinchero R, Adler Y. Risk of constrictive pericarditis after acute pericarditis. Circulation. 2011;124:1270–5.
6. Cameron J, Oesterle SN, Baldwin JC, Hancock EW. The etiologic spectrum of constrictive pericarditis. Am Heart J. 1987;113(2 Pt 1):354–80.
7. Ling LH, Oh JK, Schaff HV, Danielson GK, Mahoney DW, Seward JB, et al. Constrictive pericarditis in the modern era: evolving clinical spectrum and impact on outcome after pericardiectomy. Circulation. 1999;100:1380–6.
8. Bertog SC, Thambidorai SK, Parakh K, Schoenhagen P, Ozduran V, Houghtaling PL, et al. Constrictive pericarditis: etiology and cause-specific survival after pericardiectomy. J Am Coll Cardiol. 2004;43:1445–52.
9. Mutyaba AK, Balkaran S, Cloete R, du Plessis N, Badri M, Brink J, Mayosi BM. Constrictive pericarditis requiring pericardiectomy at Groote Schuur Hospital, Cape Town, South Africa: causes and perioperative outcomes in the HIV era (1990–2012). J Thorac Cardiovasc Surg. 2014;148:3058–65.
10. Talreja DR, Edwards WD, Danielson GK, Schaff HV, Tajik AJ, Tazelaar HD, et al. Constrictive pericarditis in 26 patients with histologically normal pericardial thickness. Circulation. 2003;108:1852–7.
11. Welch TD, Ling LH, Espinosa RE, Anavekar NS, Wiste HJ, Lahr BD, Schaff HV, Oh JK. Echocardiographic diagnosis of constrictive pericarditis: Mayo Clinic criteria. Circ Cardiovasc Imaging. 2014;7:526–34.
12. Talreja DR, Nishimura RA, Oh JK, Holmes DR. Constrictive pericarditis in the modern era: novel criteria for diagnosis in the cardiac catheterization laboratory. J Am Coll Cardiol. 2008;51:315–9.
13. Ferguson EC, Berkowitz EA. Cardiac and pericardial calcifications on chest radiographs. Clin Cardiol. 2010;65:685–94.
14. Sagrista-Sauleda J, Permanyer-Miralda G, Candell-Riera J, Angel J, Soler- Soler J. Transient cardiac constriction: an unrecognized pattern of evolution in effusive acute idiopathic pericarditis. Am J Cardiol. 1987;59:961–6.
15. Haley JH, Tajik AJ, Danielson GK, Schaff HV, Mulvagh SL, Oh JK. Transient constrictive pericarditis: causes and natural history. J Am Coll Cardiol. 2004;43:271–5.
16. Verhaert D, Gabriel RS, Johnston D, Lytle BW, Desai MY, Klein AL. The role of multimodality imaging in the management of pericardial disease. Circ Cardiovasc Imaging. 2010;3:333–43.

17. Yared K, Baggish AL, Picard MH, Hoffmann U, Hung J. Multimodality imaging of pericardial disease. J Am Coll Cardiol Img. 2010;3:650–60.
18. Syed FF, Schaff HV, Oh JK. Constrictive pericarditis--a curable diastolic heart failure. Nat Rev Cardiol. 2014;11:530–44.
19. DeValeria PA, Baumgartner WA, Casale AS, Greene PS, Cameron DE, Gardner TJ, et al. Current indications, risks, and outcome after pericardiectomy. Ann Thorac Surg. 1991;52:219–24.
20. Chowdhury UK, Subramaniam GK, Kumar AS, Airan B, Singh R, Talwar S, et al. Pericardiectomy for constrictive pericarditis: a clinical, echocardiographic, and hemodynamic evaluation of two surgical techniques. Ann Thorac Surg. 2006;81:522–9.
21. Cho YH, Schaff HV, Dearani JA, et al. Completion pericardiectomy for recurrent constrictive pericarditis: importance of timing of recurrence on late clinical outcome of operation. Ann Thorac Surg. 2012;93:1236–41.
22. Komoda T, Frumkin A, Knosalla C, Hetzer R. Child-Pugh score predicts survival after radical pericardiectomy for constrictive pericarditis. Ann Thorac Surg. 2013;96:1679–85.
23. Sagrista-Sauleda J, Angel J, Sanchez A, Permanyer-Miralda G, Soler-Soler J. Effusive-constrictive pericarditis. N Engl J Med. 2004;350:469–75.
24. Ntsekhe M, Wiysonge CS, Commerford PJ, Mayosi BM. The prevalence and outcome of effusive constrictive pericarditis: a systematic review of the literature. Cardiovasc J Afr. 2012;23:281–5.

Congenital Abnormalities of the Pericardium and Pericardial Masses

16

16.1 Classification

The pathological entities that are discussed in this chapter represent diseases that can be rarely encountered in clinical practice.

A practical, simple classification is reported in Table 16.1.

16.2 Congenital Abnormalities of the Pericardium

Congenital abnormalities of the pericardium are rare diseases in clinical practice, but often show typical abnormal imaging findings that are important to recognize.

The main congenital abnormalities of the pericardium include:

1. Pericardial defects
2. Congenital cysts

Table 16.1 Congenital disease and pericardial masses

Congenital diseases	Pericardial defects (partial or complete)
	Congenital cysts and diverticula
Pericardial masses	Tumours:
	Primary (very rare: pericardial mesothelioma in 50 % of cases)
	Secondary (common: especially lung and breast cancer, sometimes lymphomas and melanoma or invasion of contiguous cancer, e.g. oesophagus)
	Cysts:
	Congenital
	Acquired (essentially hydatid cyst in echinococcosis)
	Haematoma

© Springer International Publishing Switzerland 2016
M. Imazio, *Myopericardial Diseases: Diagnosis and Management*,
DOI 10.1007/978-3-319-27156-9_16

Pericardial Defects

Pericardial defects are rare diseases that may be partial or complete. The extension of the defect is variable and may occur anywhere but with a preference for the portion of the pericardium covering the left side of the heart [1–3].

Pericardial defects may be associated with other congenital abnormalities (e.g. atrial septal defect, patent ductus arteriosus, bicuspid aortic valve or pulmonary malformations).

Complete absence of the entire pericardium is a rare congenital anomaly that is usually asymptomatic and has no impact on survival. It is commonly an incidental finding because of secondary abnormalities on ECG (usually right axis deviation of the QRS and right bundle branch block pattern) and echocardiography caused by an abnormal motility and displacement of cardiac chambers not fixed by the pericardium as in physiologic conditions.

Displacement of cardiac chambers may simulate abnormalities of the ventricles, especially the right (e.g. arrhythmogenic right ventricular dysplasia). Pericardial defects can be well demonstrated by cardiac magnetic resonance (Fig. 16.1).

Partial defects may be dangerous since herniation of parts of the heart (such as left atrium appendage) may cause ischaemic necrosis and compression of the left coronary artery by herniation may also cause myocardial ischaemia. In these cases, surgical correction of the defect is warranted [3].

Congenital Cysts

Congenital cysts of the pericardium are rare diseases with a reported incidence of 1 in 100,000, but are the most common benign pericardial masses.

Congenital pericardial cysts are generated by the pericardium during its development and may be found anywhere in the mediastinum, but the most

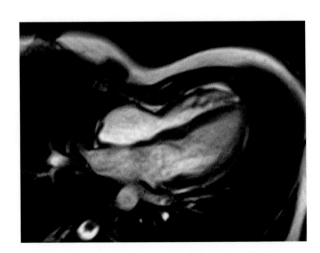

Fig. 16.1 Marked leftward displacement of the heart. The pericardium was not apparent on either side of the heart: total pericardial agenesis was diagnosed on CMR

common site is the right cardiophrenic angle. Pericardial cysts are typically located at the right cardiophrenic angle (51–70 %) or left cardiophrenic angle (28–38 %) and rarely in other mediastinal locations not adjacent to the diaphragm (8–11 %) [3].

These lesions are typically round or elliptical with a variable size of few centimetres up to >20 cm, well defined and without communication with the pericardial cavity. Histologically these cysts are lined with a single layer of mesothelial cells, with the remainder of the wall composed of connective tissue with collagen and elastic fibres. They contain a clear water-like fluid.

They are usually asymptomatic and incidental finding on imaging studies but may become symptomatic in case of complications (haemorrhage, infection): in this case they usually increase their size and may give symptoms related to their compressive effect on adjacent anatomic structures [4–6].

Congenital pericardial cysts appear as round or elliptical masses with the same density of water on CT imaging. Due to its high water content, they appear with a uniform high signal on T2-weighted images (Fig. 16.2) and usually have intermediate signal intensity on T1-weighted images. The signal may be increased on T1-weighted images if the content is highly proteinaceous. In the absence of complications (e.g. inflammation), pericardial cyst does not show contrast enhancement [1, 2, 5].

As mentioned surgery is routinely not recommended for pericardial cysts, unless symptomatic with compression of adjacent organs. However, 10 % of all cysts may be instead a *pericardial diverticulum* with a persistent connection to the pericardial space, not apparent from radiologic studies, and that can be identified only at surgery. These lesions may cause atypical symptoms that are relieved only after surgery [7]. Minimally invasive thoracoscopic resection of a pericardial cyst is a less invasive alternative option because it minimizes surgical trauma and postoperative pain and has shorter recovery period. An alternative option is percutaneous aspiration of cyst contents.

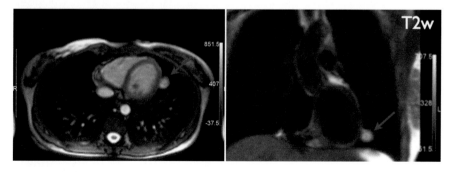

Fig. 16.2 A pericardial cyst adjacent to the left ventricle presenting an uniform high signal on T2-weighted images (see *red arrows*)

16.3   Pericardial Masses

Pericardial masses include cysts, pericardial tumours and pericardial haematomas [1, 2].

Cysts

Congenital cysts are rare and have been discussed in congenital abnormalities. Acquired cysts of the pericardium are less common. The most common cause of acquired pericardial cyst is echinococcosis. Cardiac hydatid cyst disease is uncommon, representing approximately less than 2 % of all cyst-related cases. The liver (>65 % of cases) and lungs (25 % of cases) are the most commonly involved organs in hydatid cyst disease. In cases with cardiac involvement, as the cyst reaches the myocardium either by coronary arteries (primary involvement) or by pulmonary cyst rupture in the pulmonary veins (secondary involvement), a period of 1–5 years is required for the formation of the cyst. Cardiac hydatid cysts are found mostly within the myocardium. Their most common location is in the left ventricle (50–70 % of cases), followed by the atria and the free wall of the right ventricle (30 % of cases), the pericardium (15–25 % of cases) and the interventricular septum (5–15 % of cases). Hydatid cysts of the left ventricle are usually subepicardial, whereas the right ventricle usually has subendocardial hydatid cysts [8]. Symptoms are closely related to the location and the size of the cysts. At early stages, a patient is usually asymptomatic. After the cyst reaches a significant size, some symptoms and complications can ensue. Conduction abnormalities, arrhythmias, anaphylactic shock, central or peripheral arterial embolism, pulmonary embolism and cardiac tamponade are among the serious complications associated with cardiac hydatid cysts. Chest roentgenogram can reveal cardiomegaly, mass on borders and bulging of the heart silhouette. Echocardiography, CT and CMR are useful for the detection of the cystic nature, exact anatomical location and wall calcification of the cysts. Internal septa may also be identified. Computed tomography and MRI are superior to echocardiography for the evaluation of the internal structure of the mass lesions, their relationship to adjacent tissues and coexisting pulmonary or mediastinal hydatid disease. Computed tomography is better for the wall calcification as small calcifications may sometimes be important clues for the diagnosis of a hydatid cyst. In general, on CT, uncomplicated cysts are clearly defined masses, whereas infected cysts are poorly defined masses. On CMR, a hydatid cyst is a round lesion that is hypointense on T_1-weighted images and hyperintense on T_2-weighted images. A pericyst is a reactive fibrous tissue; on T_2-weighted images, it is usually recognized with a hypointense rim.

Surgery is the main treatment even in asymptomatic patients as sudden complications can develop. Medical treatment (e.g. albendazole and mebendazole) is necessary as a supplement to surgery, especially for disseminated cases and for prophylaxis [8].

Pericardial Tumours

Pericardial tumours are uncommon as primary tumours. The most common primary tumour is *pericardial mesothelioma* that accounts for 50 % of all pericardial primary tumours. Pericardial mesothelioma is associated with asbestosis. The typical aspect is a diffuse involvement of the pericardium with irregular thickening and appearance of usually bloody pericardial effusion. Possible presentations include an isolated pericardial effusion, cardiac tamponade and constrictive pericarditis. However the imaging features are rather non-specific and biopsy is required for definite diagnosis [1, 2, 8].

Other primary tumours of the pericardium include lipoma (most common benign tumour of the pericardium), lymphoma, malignant teratomas and liposarcomas.

Secondary Tumours

Secondary tumours of the pericardium are more common. On autoptic studies, pericardial metastases are even more commonly detected than in clinical practice: about 10–15 % of patients dying for cancer have pericardial metastases. They are often small and difficult to detect. Common presentations include pericardial effusion and cardiac tamponade. Pericardial effusions are usually bloody. The most common neoplasms causing pericardial metastases include lung and breast cancer, lymphomas, melanoma and cancers of contiguous anatomic structures (e.g. oesophagus).

Pericardial metastases usually appear as nodules, masses and/or pericardial thickening on CT and CMR [1, 2, 8].

Pericardial Haematomas

Pericardial haematomas are commonly found after trauma and surgery. A recent haematoma has an initial increased attenuation that decreases over time. Chronic haematomas may present calcifications and show low signal [1, 2].

16.4   Multimodality Imaging for Pericardial Masses and Cysts

Pericardial masses represent a challenging diagnostic issue, where integrated and multimodality imaging is essential for the final diagnosis [1, 2]. The main features on echocardiography, CT and CMR are summarized in Table 16.2.

Table 16.2 Multimodality imaging of pericardial cysts and masses

	Echocardiography	CT	CMR
Congenital cysts	Round or elliptical echo-free areas	Round or elliptical masses with the same density of water on CT imaging	Uniform high signal on T2-weighted images and usually intermediate signal intensity on T1-weighted images. The signal may be increased on T1-weighted images if the content is highly proteinaceous
Pericardial metastases	Masses, irregular thickened pericardium with effusion	Masses, irregular thickened enhanced pericardium with effusion	Masses, irregular thickened enhanced pericardium with effusion
Mesothelioma	Irregular pericardial thickening, pericardial effusion. Tamponade and constriction	Irregular pericardial thickening	Irregular pericardial thickening
Lipoma	Uniform mass	Uniform masses of low attenuation	Uniform masses with high signal on T1-weighted images and low signal on fat-saturation images
Liposarcoma	Irregular mass, pericardial thickening	Non-uniform masses of low attenuation	Non-uniform masses with high signal on T1-weighted images and low signal on fat-saturation images
Fibroma	Uniform mass	Mass with soft tissue attenuation	Low signal masses on T1-weighted and T2-weighted images
Teratoma	Non-homogeneous mass	Non-homogeneous mass with possible calcification	Non-homogeneous mass that may contain fat tissue
Pericardial haematoma	Echo-dense effusion	Recent: high signal	Recent: high signal
		Old: low signal and possible calcifications	Old: low signal and possible calcifications

Key Points

- Congenital abnormalities are rare and include especially pericardial defects (partial or complete) that may be responsible for abnormal dislocation of the heart within the thoracic cavity and pericardial cysts.
- Pericardial cysts are usually congenital and are typically round or elliptical with a variable size of few centimetres up to >20 cm, well defined and without communication with the pericardial cavity.
- Pericardial cysts are usually asymptomatic and incidental finding on imaging studies but may become symptomatic in case of complications (haemorrhage, infection).
- Congenital pericardial cysts appear as round or elliptical masses with the same density of water on CT imaging. Due to its high water content, they appear with a uniform high signal on T2-weighted images.
- Pericardial tumours are uncommon as primary tumours.
- The most common primary tumour is pericardial mesothelioma. The typical aspect is a diffuse involvement of the pericardium with irregular thickening and appearance of usually bloody pericardial effusion. Possible presentations include an isolated pericardial effusion, cardiac tamponade and constrictive pericarditis. However the imaging features are rather non-specific and biopsy is required for definite diagnosis.
- Secondary tumours of the pericardium are more common. The most common neoplasms causing pericardial metastases include lung and breast cancer, lymphomas, melanoma and cancers of contiguous anatomic structures (e.g. oesophagus).
- Common presentations include pericardial effusion and cardiac tamponade. Pericardial effusions are usually bloody. Pericardial metastases usually appear as nodules, masses and/or pericardial thickening on CT and CMR.

References

1. Klein AL, Abbara S, Agler DA, Appleton CP, Asher CR, Hoit B, Hung J, Garcia MJ, Kronzon I, Oh JK, Rodriguez ER, Schaff HV, Schoenhagen P, Tan CD, White RD. American Society of Echocardiography clinical recommendations for multimodality cardiovascular imaging of patients with pericardial disease: endorsed by the Society for Cardiovascular Magnetic Resonance and Society of Cardiovascular Computed Tomography. J Am Soc Echocardiogr. 2013;26:965–1012.e15.

2. Cosyns B, Plein S, Nihoyanopoulos P, Smiseth O, Achenbach S, Andrade MJ, Pepi M, Ristic A, Imazio M, Paelinck B, Lancellotti P, On behalf of the European Association of Cardiovascular Imaging (EACVI) and European Society of Cardiology Working Group (ESC WG) on Myocardial and Pericardial diseases. European Association of Cardiovascular Imaging (EACVI) position paper: multimodality imaging in pericardial disease. Eur Heart J Cardiovasc Imaging. 2014;16:12–31.
3. Peebles CR, Shambrook JS, Harden SP. Pericardial disease – anatomy and function. Br J Radiol. 2011;84(Spec No 3):S324–37.
4. Islas F, de Agustin JA, Gomez de Diego JJ, Olmos C, Ferrera C, Luaces M, Cabeza B, Macaya C, Pérez de Isla L. Giant pericardial cyst compressing the heart. J Am Coll Cardiol. 2013;62:e19.
5. Mazhar J, Lawley C, Gill AJ, Grieve SM, Figtree GA. Visualizing pericardial inflammation as the cause of acute chest pain in a patient with a congenital pericardial cyst: the incremental diagnostic value of cardiac magnetic resonance. Eur Heart J. 2013;34:1413.
6. Nayak K, Shetty RK, Vivek G, Pai UM. Pericardial cyst: a benign anomaly. BMJ Case Rep. 2012;2012. pii: bcr0320125984.
7. Money ME, Park C. Pericardial diverticula misdiagnosed as pericardial cysts. J Thorac Cardiovasc Surg. 2015;149:e103–7.
8. Authors/Task Force Members, Adler Y, Charron P, Imazio M, Badano L, Barón-Esquivias G, Bogaert J, Brucato A, Gueret P, Klingel K, Lionis C, Maisch B, Mayosi B, Pavie A, Ristić AD, Sabaté Tenas M, Seferovic P, Swedberg K, Tomkowski W. 2015 ESC guidelines for the diagnosis and management of pericardial diseases: the task force for the diagnosis and management of pericardial diseases of the European Society of Cardiology (ESC) endorsed by: the European Association for Cardio-Thoracic Surgery (EACTS). Eur Heart J. 2015;36:2921–64.

Part III

Specific Populations, Guidelines, Conclusions and Perspectives

Age and Gender Issues in the Management of Pericardial Diseases

17

17.1 Introduction

Management of pericardial diseases should consider specific issues related to the age of patients (essentially dosing issues) and gender (especially considering specific physiological conditions such as pregnancy and lactation) [1].

17.2 Children

Pericarditis is an important cause of chest pain in children and accounts for about 5 % of all children who present with chest pain to a paediatric emergency department [2]. The aetiological spectrum has specific peculiarities since children may present more specific causes, such as bacterial, autoinflammatory diseases and especially post-pericardiotomy syndromes following surgical repair of congenital heart diseases (especially atrial septal defects) [3–5].

The same diagnostic criteria of adults apply also for pericarditis and pericardial effusions in children. However, it is typically described that children have a more marked systemic inflammatory pattern compared to adults. Fever and pleuropulmonary involvement is more commonly reported as well as elevation of markers of inflammation [5].

Unfortunately, at present, there are no RCTs in paediatric settings and thus the management of pericardial syndromes in children follows the general schemes of adults although with dose adjustments; moreover, aspirin is contraindicated in children because of the risk of Reye's syndrome (Tables 17.1 and 17.2) [1]. Colchicine can be used in children, while corticosteroid use should be restricted more than in adults, due to their possible severe side effects (striae rubre and growth impairment), which are particularly deleterious in growing children. Corticosteroid dependence is particularly critical in these patients and biological agents (e.g. anakinra) have been first used in the paediatric setting to allow corticosteroid withdrawal [6–9]. Exercise restriction is particularly bothersome for children and their

© Springer International Publishing Switzerland 2016
M. Imazio, *Myopericardial Diseases: Diagnosis and Management*,
DOI 10.1007/978-3-319-27156-9_17

Table 17.1 Dosing of non-steroidal anti-inflammatory drugs in children. Modified form 2015 ESC guidelines [1]

Drug	Dosing
Aspirin	Contraindicated in children due to the associated risk of Reye's syndrome and hepatotoxicity
Ibuprofen	30–50 mg/kg/24 h divided every 8 h; maximum: 2.4 g/day
Indomethacin	Children ≥2 years: oral, 1–2 mg/kg/day in 2–4 divided doses; maximum dose, 4 mg/kg/day; not to exceed 150–200 mg/day
Naproxen	Children >2 years: oral suspension is recommended, 10 mg/kg/day in 2 divided doses (up to 15 mg/kg/day has been tolerated); do not exceed 15 mg/kg/day

Acute pericarditis: 1–2 weeks. *Recurrent pericarditis*: several weeks. The optimal length of treatment is debatable, and C-reactive protein should be used as a marker of disease activity to guide management and treatment length. Tapering is advisable after symptom resolution and C-reactive protein normalization

Table 17.2 Colchicine dosing according to age and concomitant renal and hepatic impairment

Setting	Dose adjustment
Children:	
≤5 years	0.5 mg/day
>5 years	As for adults
Elderly (>70 years)	Reduce dose by 50 % and consider renal impairment
Renal impairment	ClCr 35–49 mL/min 0.5 mg once daily
	ClCr 10–34 mL/min 0.5 mg every 2–3 days
	ClCr <10 mL/min avoid chronic use of colchicine. Use in serious renal impairment is contraindicated by the manufacturer
Hepatic dysfunction	Avoid in severe hepatobiliary dysfunction and in patients with hepatic disease

ClCr clearance of creatinine

families, and the quality of life may be seriously affected especially in recurrent cases. Nevertheless, the prognosis is good and related to the underlying aetiology of pericardial syndromes [5].

The new 2015 ESC guidelines address the specific issue of the management of children with a pericardial syndrome [1]. Specific recommendations include:

- NSAIDs at high doses are recommended as first-line therapy for acute pericarditis in children, till complete symptom resolution (Recommendation Class I C).
- Colchicine should be considered as an adjunct to anti-inflammatory therapy for acute and recurrent pericarditis also in children, at low dosage, <5 years: 0.5 mg/day; >5 years: 1.0–1.5 mg/day in two to three divided doses (Recommendation Class IIa C).
- Anti IL1 drugs may be considered in children with recurrent pericarditis and especially when corticosteroid dependent (Recommendation Class IIb C).
- Aspirin is not recommended in children due to the associated risk of Reye's syndrome and hepatotoxicity (Recommendation Class III C).
- Corticosteroids are not recommended due to the severity of their side effects in growing children, unless there are specific indications such as autoimmune diseases (Recommendation Class III C).

The low levels of recommendations reflect the evidence based essentially on case series, retrospective reviews and experts' opinion and reviews. Although possible, it seems wise in my view, in order to improve patient compliance and reduce possible side effects, not to prescribe higher doses of colchicine in children >5 years, but instead to consider the same doses of adults (e.g. 0.5 mg BID).

17.3   Pregnancy and Lactation

During pregnancy, it is relatively common (up to 40 % of cases) to detect a mild pericardial effusion by the third trimester. The effusion is generally asymptomatic and does not require any treatment [10–13].

Pericarditis may occur and treatment should consider possible effects of medical therapy on the foetus. Generally pericarditis is viral or idiopathic and has a good prognosis with outcomes similar to those reported in the general population. In patients with previous pericarditis, it is wise to plan pregnancy in a phase of quiescence of the disease. For the medical therapy of pericarditis, aspirin and NSAIDs (ibuprofen and indomethacin) may be prescribed during the first and second trimester. After gestational week 20, all NSAIDs (except aspirin ≤ 100 mg/day) can cause constriction of the ductus arteriosus and impair foetal renal function, and they are withdrawn in any case at gestational week 32. On this basis, low-dose corticosteroids (e.g. prednisone 0.2–0.5 mg/kg/day) represent a valid option that can be adopted for the whole duration of pregnancy (Table 17.3). In the absence of a specific indication (e.g. Familial Mediterranean Fever), colchicine is considered contraindicated during pregnancy [1, 10–15].

Paracetamol is allowed throughout pregnancy and breastfeeding, as are antihistamine H2 blockers or proton pump inhibitors [16].

Normal vaginal delivery is possible and should be considered in the absence of contraindications.

During breastfeeding, ibuprofen, indomethacin, naproxen and prednisone may be considered, while colchicine is contraindicated. Colchicine is considered contraindicated during pregnancy and breastfeeding, although in women with Familial Mediterranean Fever, no adverse events on fertility, pregnancy or foetal or child development have been reported even after prolonged exposure to colchicine [1, 17–19].

Table 17.3 Recommended anti-inflammatory therapies for pericarditis during pregnancy

Drug	Pregnancy		After delivery
	<20 weeks	>20 weeks	During breastfeeding
Aspirin[a] 500–750 mg every 8 h	Possible	To be avoided	Preferably avoided
NSAID (ibuprofen, indomethacin, naproxen)	Allowed	To be avoided	Allowed
Paracetamol	Allowed	Allowed	Allowed
Prednisone low dose	Allowed	Allowed	Allowed

Possible association with aspirin or an NSAID and prednisone; prednisone is metabolized by the placenta into inactive 11-keto forms, and only 10 % of the active drugs may reach the foetus
[a]A dose of aspirin less than or equal to 100 mg/d is not useful as anti-inflammatory therapy

17.4   The Elderly

Elderly patients may be affected by all types of pericardial syndromes. The general principles of diagnosis and therapy follow those outlined for the general population. Unfortunately there are no specific studies addressing the issue of pericardial diseases in the elderly [1].

Dose adjustments should be considered with the lowest effective dose also considering the possible presence of renal impairment that is very common in these patients. A specific additional issue for the elderly is represented by therapy adherence and compliance that may be problematic in the elderly because of cognitive impairment, poor vision or hearing, number of medications and costs [20].

Specific recommendations of the 2015 ESC guidelines are to avoid indomethacin, halving doses of colchicine, and pay particular attention to the evaluation of renal impairment and drug interactions [1].

Key Points
- Unfortunately, at present, there are no RCTs in paediatric settings and thus the management of pericardial syndromes in children follows the general schemes of adults although with dose adjustments.
- Aspirin is contraindicated in children because of the risk of Reye's syndrome.
- Colchicine should be considered as an adjunct to anti-inflammatory therapy for acute recurrent pericarditis also in children, at low dosage if <5 years: 0.5 mg/day; but as for adults if >5 years.
- Corticosteroids use should be avoided as much as possible due to the severity of their side effects in growing children, unless there are specific indications.
- Anti IL1 drugs may be considered in children with recurrent pericarditis and especially when corticosteroid dependent.
- During pregnancy, the medical therapy of pericarditis may be based on aspirin and NSAIDs (ibuprofen and indomethacin) that may be prescribed during the first and second trimester. After gestational week 20, all NSAIDs (except aspirin ≤ 100 mg/day) can cause constriction of the ductus arteriosus and impair foetal renal function, and they are withdrawn in any case at gestational week 32.
- Low-dose corticosteroids (e.g. prednisone 0.2–0.5 mg/kg/day) represent a valid option that can be adopted for the whole duration of pregnancy.
- In the absence of a specific indication (e.g. Familial Mediterranean Fever), colchicine is considered contraindicated during pregnancy and lactation.
- In the elderly, dose adjustments should be considered for medical therapies also considering possible drug interactions and the presence of renal impairment that is very common in these patients.

References

1. Authors/Task Force Members, Adler Y, Charron P, Imazio M, Badano L, Barón-Esquivias G, Bogaert J, Brucato A, Gueret P, Klingel K, Lionis C, Maisch B, Mayosi B, Pavie A, Ristić AD, Sabaté Tenas M, Seferovic P, Swedberg K, Tomkowski W. 2015 ESC guidelines for the diagnosis and management of pericardial diseases: the task force for the diagnosis and management of pericardial diseases of the European Society of Cardiology (ESC) endorsed by: the European Association for Cardio-Thoracic Surgery (EACTS). Eur Heart J. 2015;36:2921–64.
2. Geggel RL. Conditions leading to pediatric cardiology consultation in a tertiary academic hospital pediatrics. Pediatrics. 2004;114:409–17.
3. Shakti D, Hehn R, Gauvreau K, Sundel RP, Newburger JW. Idiopathic pericarditis and pericardial effusion in children: contemporary epidemiology and management. J Am Heart Assoc. 2014;3, e001483.
4. Raatikka M, Pelkonem PM, Karjalainen J, Jokinen E. Recurrent pericariditis in children and adolescents. J Am Coll Cardiol. 2003;42:759–64.
5. Imazio M, Brucato A, Pluymaekers N, Breda L, Calabri G, Cantarini L, Cimaz R, Colimodio F, Corona F, Cumetti D, Di Blasi Lo Cuccio C, Gattorno M, Insalaco A, Limongelli G, Russo MG, Valenti A, Finkelstein Y, Martini A. Recurrent pericarditis in children and adolescents: etiology, presentation, therapies, and outcomes. A multicenter cohort study. J Cardiovasc Med. 2016; in press.
6. Picco P, Brisca G, Traverso F, Loy A, Gattorno M, Martini A. Successful treatment of idiopathic recurrent pericarditis in children with interleukin-1β receptor antagonist (anakinra): an unrecognized autoinflammatory disease? Arthritis Rheum. 2009;60:264–8.
7. Finetti M, Insalaco A, Cantarini L, Meini A, Breda L, Alessio M, D'Alessandro M, Picco P, Martini A, Gattorno M. Long term efficacy of interleukin-1 receptor antagonist (anakinra) in steroid dependent and colchicine-resistant recurrent pericarditis. J Pediatr. 2014;164:1425–31.
8. Scardapane A, Brucato A, Chiarelli F, Breda L. Efficacy of interleukin-1beta receptor antagonist (anakinra) in idiopathic recurrent pericarditis. Pediatr Cardiol. 2013;34:1989–91.
9. Gaspari S, Marsili M, Imazio M, Brucato A. New insights in the pathogenesis and therapy of idiopathic recurrent pericarditis in children. Clin Exp Rheumatol. 2013;31:788–94.
10. Ristić AD, Seferović PM, Ljubić A, Jovanović I, Ristić G, Pankuweit S, Ostojić M, Maisch B. Pericardial disease in pregnancy. Herz. 2003;28:209–15.
11. Brucato A, Imazio M, Curri S, Palmieri G, Trinchero R. Medical treatment of pericarditis during pregnancy. Int J Cardiol. 2010;144:413–4.
12. Imazio M, Brucato A. Management of pericarditis in women. Womens Health (Lond Engl). 2012;8:341–8.
13. Imazio M, Brucato A, Rampello S, Armellino F, Trinchero R, Spodick DH, Adler Y. Management of pericardial diseases during pregnancy. J Cardiovasc Med (Hagerstown). 2010;11:557–62.
14. Østensen M, Khamashta M, Lockshin M, Parke A, Brucato A, Carp H, Doria A, Rai R, Meroni P, Cetin I, Derksen R, Branch W, Motta M, Gordon C, Ruiz-Irastorza G, Spinillo A, Friedman D, Cimaz R, Czeizel A, Piette JC, Cervera R, Levy RA, Clementi M, De Carolis S, Petri M, Shoenfeld Y, Faden D, Valesini G, Tincani A. Anti-inflammatory and immunosuppressive drugs and reproduction. Arthritis Res Ther. 2006;8:209.
15. Henderson JT, Whitlock EP, O'Connor E, Senger CA, Thompson JH, Rowland MG. Low-dose aspirin for prevention of morbidity and mortality from preeclampsia: a systematic evidence review for the U.S. Preventive Services Task Force. Ann Intern Med. 2014;160:695–703.
16. Gill SK, O'Brien L, Einarson TR, Koren G. The safety of proton pump inhibitors (PPIs) in pregnancy: a meta-analysis. Am J Gastroenterol. 2009;104:1541–5.
17. Ben-Chetrit E, Levy M. Reproductive system in familial Mediterranean fever: an overview. Ann Rheum Dis. 2003;62:916–9.

18. Ben-Chetrit E, Scherrmann JM, Levy M. Colchicine in breast milk of patients with familial Mediterranean fever. Arthritis Rheum. 1996;39:1213–7.
19. Ehrenfeld M, Brzezinski A, Levy M, Eliakim M. Fertility and obstetric history in patients with familial Mediterranean fever on long-term colchicine therapy. Br J Obstet Gynaecol. 1987;94:1186–91.
20. Pasina L, Brucato AL, Falcone C, Cucchi E, Bresciani A, Sottocorno M, Taddei GC, Casati M, Franchi C, Djade CD, Nobili A. Medication non-adherence among elderly patients newly discharged and receiving polypharmacy. Drugs Aging. 2014;31:283–9.

Guidelines on the Management of Pericardial Diseases

18

18.1 Overview and Introduction

Consensus documents have been developed by the American Society of Echocardiography, American College of Cardiology (ACC) and American Heart Association (AHA) as well as from the European Association of Cardiovascular Imaging on multimodality imaging of pericardial diseases [1, 2].

Both documents are consistent and provide an overview of the main diagnostic techniques with a special focus on echocardiography, computed tomography (CT) and cardiac magnetic resonance (CMR). Strengths and weaknesses are reviewed as well as the indications and specific findings in pericardial syndromes.

An additional position paper of the working group of myocardial and pericardial diseases addresses the triage of cardiac tamponade [3]. The position paper is essentially focused on the identification of patients who need immediate drainage of the pericardial effusion, the issue of guidance of pericardiocentesis either by echocardiography or fluoroscopy and selection criteria for the transfer to specialized/tertiary institution or surgical service.

The triage system is especially created on the basis of experts' opinion and there is a need for a validation by additional prospective studies before it can be introduced and implemented in clinical practice.

National guidelines on the management of pericardial diseases have been also issued by the Spanish Society of Cardiology in 2000 [4] and more recently by the Brazilian Society of Cardiology in 2014 [5].

The first international guidelines on the management of pericardial diseases have been issued in 2004 by the European Society of Cardiology (ESC) [6]. However new important data have become available in the last 10 years, and new guidelines have been issued in 2015 by the ESC [7]. At present, there are no guidelines issued by the ACC/AHA.

© Springer International Publishing Switzerland 2016
M. Imazio, *Myopericardial Diseases: Diagnosis and Management*,
DOI 10.1007/978-3-319-27156-9_18

18.2   What's New in Pericardial Diseases?

First of all new diagnostic strategies have been proposed for the triage of patients with pericarditis and pericardial effusion and allow the selection of high-risk patients to be admitted as well as when and how additional diagnostic investigations are to be performed. Moreover specific clinical diagnostic criteria have been proposed for acute and recurrent pericarditis in clinical practice [8].

As mentioned, multimodality imaging for pericardial diseases has become an essential approach for a modern and comprehensive diagnostic evaluation, and this emerging diagnostic approach is now acknowledged, including the role of the detection of pericardial inflammation by imaging (CT/CMR) for the diagnosis of potentially reversible form of new-onset constrictive pericarditis [1, 2, 8].

The aetiology and pathophysiology of pericardial diseases remain to be better characterized, but new data supporting the immune-mediated pathogenesis of recurrences and new forms related to auto-inflammatory diseases have been documented, especially in paediatric patients.

The first prospective cohort studies have been performed on the prognosis and outcomes of acute pericarditis and myopericarditis. First epidemiological data have become available from retrospective studies on hospitalized patients.

Major advances have occurred in therapy with the first multicentre randomized clinical trials especially focused on the use of colchicine as adjunct to conventional anti-inflammatory therapies for the treatment and prevention of pericarditis.

Specific therapeutic dosing without a loading dose and weight-adjusted doses have been proposed to improve patient compliance.

Recurrences are the most troublesome complication of pericarditis, and new therapeutic choices have become available for refractory recurrent pericarditis, including alternative immunosuppressive therapies (e.g. azathioprine), iv immunoglobulins (IVIG) and interleukin-1 (IL-1) antagonists (e.g. anakinra). In these patients, also the role of pericardiectomy has been clarified as the last therapeutic option after failure of medical therapy.

In conclusion, significant new data has become available since 2004, and a new version of guidelines has become mandatory for clinical practice [7, 8].

18.3   How 2015 ESC Guidelines Are Structured and Main Messages

The 2015 ESC guidelines [7] are divided into five main parts:

1. Brief overview and introduction with a list of the aetiologies
2. A description of the main pericardial syndromes (acute and recurrent pericarditis, pericardial effusion, cardiac tamponade and constrictive pericarditis)
3. Specific forms according to the aetiology (viral pericarditis, tuberculous pericarditis, purulent pericarditis, pericardial diseases in renal failure, systemic inflammatory diseases, post-cardiac injury syndromes, traumatic pericardial effusion and haemopericardium, neoplastic pericardial diseases and other forms)

4. A brief overview of age and gender issues in the management of pericardial diseases
5. A final part on interventional techniques and surgery for pericardial diseases

In the field of pericardial diseases, there are a limited number of randomized controlled trials. Therefore, the number of Class I Level A indications is limited. The 2015 ESC guidelines are essentially clinical practice guidelines to improve and guide the management of pericardial diseases [7, 8].

On this basis, they provide definitions and diagnostic criteria and practical management issues. The present book incorporates all the new recommendations.

The main new recommendations [7] can be grouped into the following categories:

1. *Management of acute and recurrent pericarditis*:
    1. A triage is recommended to identify high-risk patients that should be admitted to hospital. Low-risk patients can be managed as outpatient (Class I, LOE B).
    2. Colchicine is now a first choice drug to be used as adjunct to aspirin/NSAID or corticosteroids in order to treat and prevent pericarditis either in acute or recurrent pericarditis (weight-adjusted doses are recommended without a loading dose, e.g. 0.5 mg BID for 3 months in acute pericarditis and 6 months in recurrent pericarditis; colchicine should be given only 0.5 mg once for patients <70 kg) (Class I, LOE A).
    3. Corticosteroids should not be prescribed as first choice in patients with acute pericarditis since they may favour chronicization (Class III, LOE C).
    4. Levels of C-reactive protein are useful to guide the treatment duration and assess the response to treatment in acute and recurrent pericarditis: anti-inflammatory therapy should be maintained till symptom resolution and C-reactive protein normalization (Class IIa, LOE C).
2. *Management and therapy of pericardial effusion*:
    1. The essential indications to drain a pericardial effusion include (I) cardiac tamponade (therapeutic pericardiocentesis), (II) a suspicion of bacterial or neoplastic aetiology, (III) persistent moderate to large pericardial effusion without response to medical therapy (Class I, LOE C).
    2. A triage system is proposed also for the management of pericardial effusion and essentially based on (I) recognize cardiac tamponade and possible bacterial of neoplastic aetiologies, (II) exclude concomitant pericarditis or treat as pericarditis, (III) identify associated underlying diseases, (IV) if chronic and large (>20 mm) consider pericardial drainage to prevent cardiac tamponade during follow-up. (Class I, LOE C).
    3. Treatment of pericardial effusions should be tailored as much as possible to the underlying aetiology (Class I, LOE C).
3. *Diagnosis and therapy of constrictive pericarditis*:
    1. CT and CMR are indicated for the evaluation of a suspected constrictive pericarditis as second-level imaging techniques after echocardiography (Class I, LOE C).

2. Cardiac catheterization is indicated only in complex cases when non-invasive imaging does not provide a clear-cut diagnosis or provides conflicting results (Class I, LOE C).
3. The mainstay of therapy for chronic constriction is radical pericardiectomy, but the need to assess the possible presence of pericardial inflammation (e.g. elevation of C-reactive protein, pericardial inflammation on CT/CMR) as precipitating cause in new-onset cases in order to treat with empiric anti-inflammatory therapy is acknowledged (Class I, LOE C).
4. *Diagnostic work-up of pericardial diseases*:
    1. First diagnostic evaluation in a patient with a clinical suspicion of pericardial disease should include focused history and physical examination, ECG, chest x-ray and routine blood tests including markers of myocardial inflammation and lesion, and renal function (Class I, LOE C).
    2. Echocardiography is the first, essential diagnostic imaging tool, while CT and CMR are second-level imaging techniques for specific indications (Class I, LOE C).
    3. Additional diagnostic testing should be targeted and clinically guided (Class I, LOE C).
5. *Management of tuberculous pericarditis and pericardial effusion*:
    1. Empiric anti-tuberculous therapy is only recommended in countries where tuberculosis is endemic and the disease is highly probable in the setting of a patient with pericarditis and pericardial effusion (Class I, LOE C).
    2. In cases with established diagnosis of tuberculous pericarditis, standard anti-tuberculous therapy is recommended for 6 months and prevents the evolution towards constrictive pericarditis (Class I, LOE C).
    3. In patients with tuberculous pericarditis with features of constriction and not responding to anti-tuberculous therapy, pericardiectomy is recommended after 4–8 weeks of medical therapy.
6. *Management of neoplastic pericardial diseases*:
    1. The definite diagnosis of neoplastic pericardial disease relies on the evidence of neoplastic cells on cytology of pericardial fluid (Class I, LOE B).
    2. Pericardial biopsy should be considered for the final aetiological diagnosis in selected cases (Class IIa, LOE B).
    3. Tumour markers in pericardial fluid may be helpful to differentiate a benign vs. a malignant pericardial effusion (Class IIa, LOE B).
    4. In cases with a confirmed diagnosis of neoplastic pericardial disease, systemic antineoplastic treatment is indicated (Class I, LOE B).
    5. Extended pericardial drainage is recommended to prevent recurrent cardiac tamponade and pericardial effusion and to provide a way for intrapericardial therapy (Class I, LOE B).
    6. Intrapericardial therapy with cytostatic agents should be considered to treat neoplastic pericardial disease (Class IIa, LOE B).

Key Points

- Consensus documents have been developed by the American Society of Echocardiography, American College of Cardiology (ACC) and American Heart Association (AHA) as well as from the European Association of Cardiovascular Imaging on multimodality imaging of pericardial diseases.
- The first international guidelines on the management of pericardial diseases have been issued in 2004 by the European Society of Cardiology (ESC). However, new important data have become available in the last 10 years, and new guidelines have been issued in 2015 by the ESC. At present, there are no guidelines issued by the ACC/AHA.
- The 2015 ESC guidelines are divided into five main parts: (1) classification and aetiology, (2) main pericardial syndromes, (3) specific aetiologies, (4) age and gender issues and (5) interventional techniques and cardiac surgery.
- In the field of pericardial diseases, there are a limited number of randomized controlled trials. Therefore, the number of Class I Level A indications is limited, and most recommendations are based on experts opinion (Level C).
- The 2015 ESC guidelines are essentially clinical practice guidelines to improve and guide the management of pericardial diseases.

References

1. Klein AL, Abbara S, Agler DA, Appleton CP, Asher CR, Hoit B, Hung J, Garcia MJ, Kronzon I, Oh JK, Rodriguez ER, Schaff HV, Schoenhagen P, Tan CD, White RD. American Society of Echocardiography clinical recommendations for multimodality cardiovascular imaging of patients with pericardial disease: endorsed by the Society for Cardiovascular Magnetic Resonance and Society of Cardiovascular Computed Tomography. J Am Soc Echocardiogr. 2013;26:965–1012.e15.
2. Cosyns B, Plein S, Nihoyanopoulos P, Smiseth O, Achenbach S, Andrade MJ, Pepi M, Ristic A, Imazio M, Paelinck B, Lancellotti P, On behalf of the European Association of Cardiovascular Imaging (EACVI) and European Society of Cardiology Working Group (ESC WG) on Myocardial and Pericardial diseases. European Association of Cardiovascular Imaging (EACVI) position paper: multimodality imaging in pericardial disease. Eur Heart J Cardiovasc Imaging. 2014;16:12–31.
3. Ristić AD, Imazio M, Adler Y, Anastasakis A, Badano LP, Brucato A, Caforio AL, Dubourg O, Elliott P, Gimeno J, Helio T, Klingel K, Linhart A, Maisch B, Mayosi B, Mogensen J, Pinto Y, Seggewiss H, Seferović PM, Tavazzi L, Tomkowski W, Charron P. Triage strategy for urgent management of cardiac tamponade: a position statement of the European Society of Cardiology Working Group on Myocardial and Pericardial Diseases. Eur Heart J. 2014;35:2279–84.

4. Sagristá Sauleda J, Almenar Bonet L, Angel Ferrer J, Bardají Ruiz A, Bosch Genover X, Guindo Soldevila J, Mercé Klein J, Permanyer Miralda C, Tello de Meneses Becerra R. The clinical practice guidelines of the Sociedad Española de Cardiología on pericardial pathology. Rev Esp Cardiol. 2000;53:394–412.
5. Montera MW, Mesquita ET, Colafranceschi AS, Oliveira Jr Jr AC, Rabischoffsky A, Ianni BM, Rochitte CE, Mady C, Mesquita CT, Azevedo CF, Bocchi EA, Saad EB, Braga FG, Fernandes F, Ramires FJ, Bacal F, Feitosa GS, Figueira HR, Souza Neto JD, Moura LA, Campos LA, Bittencourt MI, Barbosa Mde M, Moreira Mda C, Higuchi Mde L, Schwartzmann P, Rocha RM, Pereira SB, Mangini S, Martins SM, Bordignon S, Salles VA, Sociedade Brasileira de Cardiologia. I Brazilian guidelines on myocarditis and pericarditis. Arq Bras Cardiol. 2013;100(4 Suppl 1):1–36.
6. Maisch B, Seferović PM, Ristić AD, Erbel R, Rienmüller R, Adler Y, Tomkowski WZ, Thiene G, Yacoub MH, Task Force on the Diagnosis and Management of Pericardial Diseases of the European Society of Cardiology. Guidelines on the diagnosis and management of pericardial diseases executive summary; The Task force on the diagnosis and management of pericardial diseases of the European Society of Cardiology. Eur Heart J. 2004;25:587–610.
7. Authors/Task Force Members, Adler Y, Charron P, Imazio M, Badano L, Barón-Esquivias G, Bogaert J, Brucato A, Gueret P, Klingel K, Lionis C, Maisch B, Mayosi B, Pavie A, Ristić AD, Sabaté Tenas M, Seferovic P, Swedberg K, Tomkowski W. 2015 ESC guidelines for the diagnosis and management of pericardial diseases: the task force for the diagnosis and management of pericardial diseases of the European Society of Cardiology (ESC) endorsed by: the European Association for Cardio-Thoracic Surgery (EACTS). Eur Heart J. 2015;36:2921–64.
8. Imazio M, Brucato A, Badano L, Charron P, Adler Y. What's new in 2015 ESC guidelines for the management of pericardial diseases. J Cardiovasc Med. 2016; in press.

Conclusions

19

Pericardial diseases are relatively common diseases that may affect the pericardium either as an isolated disease or often as an involvement in a systemic or underlying disease. In this setting, pericardial disease may be the first manifestation of this underlying entity.

The history and clinical presentation are essential to develop a rationale, cost-effective diagnostic and management plan.

Many findings (e.g. signs, symptoms, basic instrumental data from ECG and chest x-ray) may be non-specific and thus should be appropriately integrated into the clinical evaluation.

Echocardiography is the first-level imaging technique for all patients with a suspicion of pericardial disease, while computed tomography (CT) and cardiac magnetic resonance (CMR) should be reserved for selected cases.

Although the causes of pericardial diseases are varied, they are similarly manifested in typical "pericardial syndromes" (pericarditis, pericardial effusion, cardiac tamponade, constrictive pericarditis and pericardial masses).

An epidemiological approach to the aetiological diagnosis is essential to avoid useless and expensive tests that may have limited diagnostic and therapeutic impact.

Tuberculosis is the most common cause of pericardial diseases all over the world, and this should be considered everywhere since immigration may change the aetiological spectrum of pericardial diseases even in developed countries with a current low prevalence of tuberculosis.

Nevertheless, the clinician should essentially rule out bacterial, neoplastic aetiologies and forms related to autoimmune or systemic inflammatory diseases.

Fortunately, clinical features at presentation may be very helpful to orientate the clinicians. Patients with a subacute onset, high fever >38 °C, large pericardial effusions or cardiac tamponade have usually a non-viral aetiology and more complications during follow-up. They are high-risk patients to be admitted to hospital and aetiology search is warranted for them with a special focus on bacterial and neoplastic aetiologies. In these cases, the definite diagnosis is based on the demonstration of the aetiological agent in pericardial fluid or tissue. Nevertheless, a probable

© Springer International Publishing Switzerland 2016
M. Imazio, *Myopericardial Diseases: Diagnosis and Management*,
DOI 10.1007/978-3-319-27156-9_19

diagnosis can be supported by the concomitant presence of the disease elsewhere and pericarditis/pericardial effusion (e.g. pulmonary tuberculosis and pericarditis/pericardial effusion), or biological markers correlated with the disease in pericardial fluid (e.g. adenosine deaminase or interferon gamma in pericardial fluid for tuberculous pericarditis and tumour markers in pericardial fluid for neoplastic pericardial disease).

For patients without high-risk features, outpatient management is safe and cost-effective.

The mainstay of medical therapy for viral and idiopathic forms as well as those associated with systemic inflammatory diseases or post-cardiac injury syndromes is aspirin or an NSAID plus colchicine. Corticosteroids are a second option for those with hypersensitivity to aspirin/NSAID or failure of these drugs, or specific indications (e.g. pregnancy, patients with rheumatic conditions already on corticosteroids).

If used, low to moderate doses are warranted (e.g. prednisone 0.2–0.5 mg/kg/day) with slow tapering after remission. The exact length of therapy is not well known but can be individualized maintaining the attack dose till symptom resolution and normalization of markers of inflammation. Tapering should be also considered to decrease the recurrence risk.

Recurrences are the more common and troublesome complications after pericarditis and occur in 20–30 % of cases. Other complications are especially related to the underlying aetiology. For instance, the risk of developing constriction is very low for viral/idiopathic forms, intermediate for immune-mediated forms and neoplastic aetiologies, and high for bacterial aetiologies.

Pericardial effusions are also very common but are often associated with pericarditis or an underlying disease (e.g. systemic inflammatory disease, renal failure, hypothyroidism). Chronic large effusions (>20 mm) may progress to cardiac tamponade in case of precipitating events (e.g. pericarditis and trauma), and pericardial drainage should be considered for the prevention of this complication according to the patient's will and local expertise.

Constrictive pericarditis is the final common destination of several entities. If chronic, the only definite therapy is radical pericardiectomy but transient forms may occur in recent onset forms when pericardial inflammation is present. Detection of systemic inflammation (e.g. elevation of C-reactive protein) or pericardial inflammation on an imaging technique (e.g. CT or CMR) may allow to identify those potentially reversible cases and empiric anti-inflammatory therapy is warranted.

Congenital and pericardial masses are relatively rare conditions in clinical practice.

Each patient should receive a tailored diagnostic approach according to history and clinical presentation, and therapy should be targeted at the aetiology as much as possible, although it is often empiric in a real world clinical setting. Each diagnostic method should be considered into the context of its clinical implications, since it may be expensive and may carry potential risks (e.g. interventional techniques) and it is clinically meaningful only if it can affect or change the clinical management.

Perspectives and Unmet Needs

20

Despite a large amount of new data, there are still several questions looking for a reply.

The aetiology and pathophysiology of pericardial disease is still not well known, especially in conditions, such as recurrent pericarditis, that are challenging and require new diagnostic and therapeutic tools to improve the management and reduce its incidence.

Even for established therapies, such as empiric anti-inflammatory therapy of pericarditis, the best duration of therapy is not clear and if tapering may be helpful to improve the outcomes.

The role of non-pharmacological measures is also controversial. Exercise restriction is usually recommended in patients with inflammatory pericardial and myopericardial syndromes, but it is unclear if it is really necessary in all cases and what is the appropriate duration of the physical restriction, especially when apparent clinical remission is achieved.

New therapies are needed to improve the outcomes in specific conditions, such as the prevention of recurrent and constrictive pericarditis, and the treatment of tuberculous pericarditis.

The exact relationship between pericarditis and myocarditis is not well known, as well as the best management of myopericarditis and the prognostic meaning of persistent late gadolinium enhancement in those patients, as reasonable evidence of myocardial fibrosis (it is unknown the possible arrhythmic risk, possible long-term evolution in ventricular dysfunction, cardiomyopathy).

Isolated pericardial effusions are a common finding in clinical practice but still not well understood in terms of aetiology, therapy, and prognosis.

The role of interventional techniques for the diagnosis and therapy is still to be well defined as well as intrapericardial therapies.

Pericardiectomy is emerging as a potential therapeutic option for recurrent inflammatory pericardial syndromes, but there are no prospective studies to support this indication beyond constrictive pericarditis, and there is a need for more centres with experience in this type of surgery.

© Springer International Publishing Switzerland 2016
M. Imazio, *Myopericardial Diseases: Diagnosis and Management*,
DOI 10.1007/978-3-319-27156-9_20

Pericardial diseases have been the "Cinderella" of heart diseases for decades. They are poorly understood and studied even in medical schools, but not so uncommon in clinical practice, and often complex to manage since they are affecting several medical specialties (cardiology, cardiac surgery, internal medicine, pulmonary medicine, infectious diseases, immunology, rheumatology, nephrology and oncology). Fortunately, the story is changing and there is growing interest on the diagnosis and therapy and first prospective and randomized clinical trials.

However, although pericardial diseases are now more on the road of evidence-based medicine than 10 years ago, there is still a long way to go and need for additional basic science and clinical studies to improve the diagnosis, therapy and prognosis of pericardial diseases in the future years.